PENGUIN

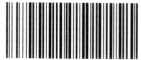

CHANGING HABITS
CHANGING LIVES

Not your typical nutritionist, Cyndi O'Meara disagrees with low-fat and low-calorie diets, believes chocolate can be good for you, and thinks cheating and eating yummy food are important parts of a well-balanced diet. Cyndi must be doing something right because she maintains a healthy weight and has never in her life taken an antibiotic, painkiller or any other form of medication.

The author of two bestselling books, *Changing Habits Changing Lives* and the accompanying *Changing Habits Changing Lives Cookbook*, Cyndi is in high demand nationally and internationally as a keynote speaker.

A lively and inspiring health expert and lifestyle coach, Cyndi has regularly appeared on national talkback radio, writes frequently for magazines and newspapers, and has shared her tips with audiences of such television programs as *Today Tonight*, *Brisbane Extra*, *Fresh*, *Peak Health and Fitness* and the forthcoming *Nourish*.

Her qualifications include a Bachelor of Science degree majoring in Nutrition from Deakin University and the University of Colorado in Boulder, Colorado, as well as postgraduate studies in human anatomy, pathology and physiology, and diplomas in diagnosis and management of health issues. Cyndi was named Sunshine Coast Business Women of the Year in 2003.

To my Mum,
my greatest teacher,
Janet Elizabeth Lovett
1937 – 2006
and to my Sister,
Lisa Anne Lovett,
my greatest mentor
1959 – 2007

CHANGING Habits CHANGING Lives

CYNDI O'MEARA

PENGUIN BOOKS

It is recommended that all individuals seek professional medical advice before making any changes to their diet. The ideas, information and suggestions in this book are purely those of the author and are not substitutes for consulting with your physician. The author and the publisher will not accept responsibility for any action or claim resulting from the use of information contained in this book.

PENGUIN BOOKS

Published by the Penguin Group
Penguin Group (Australia)
250 Camberwell Road, Camberwell, Victoria 3124, Australia
(a division of Pearson Australia Group Pty Ltd)
Penguin Group (USA) Inc.
375 Hudson Street, New York, New York 10014, USA
Penguin Group (Canada)
90 Eglinton Avenue East, Suite 700, Toronto ON M4P 2Y3, Canada
(a division of Pearson Penguin Canada Inc.)
Penguin Books Ltd
80 Strand, London WC2R 0RL, England
Penguin Ireland
25 St Stephen's Green, Dublin 2, Ireland
(a division of Penguin Books Ltd)
Penguin Books India Pvt Ltd
11 Community Centre, Panchsheel Park, New Delhi – 110 017, India
Penguin Group (NZ)
67 Apollo Drive, Rosedale, North Shore 0632, New Zealand
(a division of Pearson New Zealand Ltd)
Penguin Books (South Africa) (Pty) Ltd
24 Sturdee Avenue, Rosebank, Johannesburg 2196, South Africa

Penguin Books Ltd, Registered Offices: 80 Strand, London, WC2R 0RL, England

First published by Oracle Press, 1998
This revised edition published by Penguin Group (Australia), 2007

9 10

Cover design © Penguin Group (Australia)
Illustrations by Michelle Katsouranis
Cover photograph by Michael Paul, Getty Images
Author photograph by Starshots
Typeset in 10.5/15.5pt New Caledonia by Post Pre-press Group, Brisbane, Queensland
Printed and bound in Australia by McPherson's Printing Group, Maryborough, Victoria

National Library of Australia
Cataloguing-in-Publication data:
O'Meara, Cyndi.
Changing habits, changing lives.
Includes index.
ISBN: 978 0 14 300652 7 (pbk).
1. Health. 2. Food habits. 3. Diet. I. Title.
613.7

penguin.com.au

ACKNOWLEDGEMENTS

Life is shaped by the people you meet and the places you go. Words and actions shape the way we think and act in life. It may have been just a word or an action that took me to my next stage in life. It may have been a brief encounter or a long friendship that has shaped the way I think and act. I'd like to thank everyone I've met throughout my life for contributing in some way to where I am today.

Specifically for where my life started, I'd like to thank my Mum and Dad, Janet and David Lovett, two amazing individuals who were always positive and encouraging with every step of my life and continue to be my biggest advocates. My sister Lisa Lovett who for the last forty-six years has been my mentor and sounding board; whenever I had a tough question she always came up with an easy answer which seemed to elude me. My brother Marcus Lovett, the most wonderful brother I could ask for; so full of fun, enthusiasm and zest, you can't help but be caught up in his love of life.

Between leaving my first family and starting my own there were many people along the road that influenced my next step in life. My high school teachers from Saint Mary's College Bendigo, Sister Carmel, Mrs Peoples and Mr Kennedy. Katie Felicia, a woman who made the statement, "You're a smart girl, you're not going to waste that talent doing nothing", and who then sent me on a journey of self-discovery, taking me far from family and friends and into a country and world that really put me on this path. The result was that I attended the University of Colorado in Boulder and was taught by the most amazing man, who gave me a passion for diet and anthropology, my anthropology professor, Dennis Van Gervan. You have no idea how profound you were in my life and I failed to tell you.

Of course, my family have been my greatest influence. My patient husband of twenty years, Howard, a man of many talents who pushes me every day of my life to strive to be the best. My beautiful stepdaughter Fran Lietke, who defies the word 'step'; she is always there for me when I need her with her big heart and kind words. My son Brogan, a young man with amazing inner strength which he is still yet to realize. My gorgeous, profound daughter Casie, who teaches me so much and is wise beyond her years. And last, but not least, my loving, beautiful daughter Tarnea, the strongest and most determined of them all. Thank you for being in my life and being the reason why I do what I do.

There are many people and associations along the way that have helped me get to here right now. My dear friend, Anna Kurz Rogers, is always there for me. My wonderful friend, sounding board and walking partner Rikki Latcham and ex walking partner Cassie Sherman, who came up with the name of this book. To Mark, Jacki, Ali, Stefan and Jason Postles, a family that continues to influence many things I do. High school friends Anne Carter, Kathy McKern, Liz Johnson, Julie Mulqueen, Dobby, Amanda Griffin, Michelle and Andrew Douglas, and Gabriel McLean (our chance meeting in WA still holds a special place in my life). Current and past friends who have had insightful influences like Andrea Lynch, Chris Ezzy, Chris Cameron, Natalie Cook, Sarah Maxwell, Jenny Johnson, Jodie McIver, Kathy Ledger, Meegan Chatham, Leslie Grace, Kay Nuissl, Kim Morrison, Rachael Bermingham, Carol Robertson, Sue Maitland, Christina Glucina,

Cherry Rosenberg, Fleur Whelligan, Kerri Brooker, Catherine Henderson, Andrea and Greg Marslen, Irene O'Brien, Suzanne and Peter Snodgrass, Wayne and Angela Todd, Peter and Rita Marshal, Mark and Sioban Steven, Nym Kim, the Dennis Family, Jeremy and Kate Atkins, Jenny and Mike Jeffreys, Kerri and Ross Morey, Jeannette Martin, Tina Jacobson, Tracey Kennedy, the Floreani family, the Barham Family, Denise Smith, Lisa Clark, Ray and Connie Henderson, Virginia Anderson, Trent, Natalie Cook, Lisa Curry-Kenny, the late great Steve Irwin and inspirational wife Terri. And, not to forget family members: my sister-in-law Suzannah Petty; my mother-in-law Betty O'Meara; Kevin, Margaret and Wendy O'Meara; Mary and Patrick Kearney; Clare White, Judy Kerby, Steve Goedken and their families; as well as the Lovett clan. Thank you for what you have added to my life.

I'd like to also thank all the clients who have trusted and taken the leap of faith to create health and wellbeing in their individual lives and organisations.

To the people who have worked on this manuscript from the beginning: Stewart Forge, Angie Snaith, Suzanne Dean, Michael Nolan and other editors at Penguin Australia. And a special thank you to Robert Sessions and Graeme Morrison from Penguin.

CONTENTS

A NOTE FROM CYNDI O'MEARA

I went to an all-girl's school in the 60s and 70s. There were around 600 students at the school and I only remember one girl being overweight. At the tuckshop during recess and lunch we were able to buy meat pies, chocolate éclairs, vanilla slices, donuts, hot chips, etc. On our way home from school, we would walk to the local fish and chip shop and buy twenty cents worth of hot chips and sprinkle them with salt and vinegar. No one seemed to have a weight problem.

Why is it that we could do that then, but now children eat similar foods and there is an obesity epidemic? Inactivity is not the culprit – it is the fundamental ingredients of the food that we eat now, which were not in our foods then, that has created an epidemic of lifestyle diseases.

Changing Habits Changing Lives has been important in teaching people about healthy lifestyle and dietary choices and the changes that have occurred in the last thirty years to the ingredients of what we eat. The food may look the same but the ingredients have been technologically changed. Instead of butter we have hydrogenated vegetable oil with trans fats; instead of cocoa there is cocoa flavouring and brown colouring; instead of real cream, it's fake; instead of real eggs in the custard of a vanilla slice it is a powder; meat pies are no longer all meat; and pastry is no longer made with just a few simple ingredients. To understand this phenomenal change is to understand the path back to real food and good health.

Every year the food industry comes up with more new technology foods and it is important that the consumer is informed about their ill effects. I've now added eleven new chapters to the original 1998 edition of *Changing Habits Changing Lives* to keep you abreast of food changes over the past eight years. When I first wrote about many natural foods they were not readily available, but it is wonderful that now, as people are realising that foods from nature rather than technology are the key to health and wellbeing, the demand for these foods has made them available in many grocery and specialty stores: foods like unadulterated real milk and cream, organic flour, rapadura sugar, organic free-range eggs, real juices, and many more. There is a plethora of healthy foods and there are no more excuses.

If you're a new reader, enjoy the freedom this book will give you, with revitalised health and energy. If you're a trusted follower of *Changing Habits Changing Lives*, the new information in this updated edition will spur you on to continue your quest for healthy living.

Happy Changing Habits!

THE BEGINNING

You're probably thinking, 'Oh no, another diet book!' You may have tried other books, with no great success. Is this one different? Well, believe it or not, it is. It's not about attaining the physique of a supermodel or top athlete; it's about rediscovering the good health and high energy levels that your body is capable of producing when it receives the proper fuel.

Nearly every diet book over the past 25 years has been about 'how much'. How many calories can you consume? How many grams of protein can you eat? How much bread? What percentage of fat? This is not about how much, although there are guidelines. This eating program is about the *quality* of the food you eat rather than the *quantity*. When the quality of your food is good, then the quantity issue takes care of itself. The body is a marvellous tool – it has the capacity to tell you when you've had enough. But more on that later.

This is not a *revolutionary* diet, like the high protein diet or the low fat diet. It's an *evolutionary* diet. It is not something new – it's something quite old. In fact this way of eating has been around for thousands of years, and has stood the test of time. With this diet the human race has slowly evolved into the species we are today. As a consequence, this is a diet which our bodies thrive on.

But forty or fifty years ago, something changed. This was the beginning of what was termed the information age, when for the first time people became more interested in nourishing their brain with information and less worried about what they fed their bodies. This was the beginning of the takeaway age; fast foods, new technologies, genetically modified foods and the introduction of thousands of never-before-seen chemicals into our food chain. Since then, many new health problems have reared their ugly heads.

Many of the ailments that afflict people in our modern society are related to our lifestyle and all the trimmings that go with it. The three major diseases of the western world are heart disease, cancer and diabetes. They either kill you or put you in hospital. And once you're in hospital the risks continue. Hospital mishaps are now Australia's third biggest killer or cause of disability, and they are the biggest cause of death in the USA, followed by heart disease and cancer. These deaths and disabilities are largely unrelated to the original illness. The majority of the deaths are either a result of infections, a hospital procedure gone wrong, or reactions to prescribed medications.

The aim of a healthy diet is to prevent disease, and to keep you out of hospital and away from the medicine cabinet. The body is extremely resilient and, given the right treatment and conditions, can recuperate from many major illnesses. But taking that attitude is a little like shutting the stable door after the horse has bolted. It is much better to do everything in your power to stay healthy and try to avoid illness in the first place.

Beside the killer illnesses there are common ailments which seem to affect many people these days. Everyone seems to be tired. Chronic fatigue syndrome is the latest term to describe health problems that seem to have no cause. My opinion is that there is no single culprit for this mystery ailment, but rather a multitude of factors including poor diet, very little exercise, an unhealthy lifestyle, and a concentration of drugs and chemicals in our food chain and environment.

A healthy diet is not just about the number of calories or the amount of fat; it should take a holistic approach. This book is also about changing your lifestyle, the way you feel, the way you think about food, and how you respond to other people. An unhealthy person is usually an unhappy person. This diet is about gaining health, energy, vitality and, consequently, happiness. If you also lose weight, then that's a bonus from being healthy. After all, wouldn't you rather make it your goal to gain health rather than to lose weight? It's far more productive to gain something.

We are all individuals with different needs, and this diet accommodates that fact as much as possible. No single diet will suit every person, and there is a good reason for that, as you will discover later in this book. The main thread of the diet is the link between human evolution and our eating habits. As you read further you will gain an education about food, rather than a rigid regime of what to eat, how much to eat, how many calories to consume and how much exercise to do. By reading this book you will learn about food – what is done to processed foods, what additives do to foods and our bodies, and the consequences of eating different foods. With this knowledge, you can make educated choices about what to eat.

Change is one of the scariest things to do – people like to sit in their comfort zone and continue the habits they have because it takes less energy. To make changes will require energy and commitment. Many people make changes in their lives in times of crisis. If there is a health crisis, it motivates people to change. Before reading on, I'd like you to sit and contemplate your answer to the following question: If you were told that you had a fatal disease and the only way you could survive was to change your lifestyle, would you do it?

Just about everyone answers a resounding 'Yes!' But the reality of what follows is quite different, as research shows. Most people will change, but after a week it is all too hard and they revert back to their old ways. The statistics tell us that only one in ten people will change when give this ultimatum to save their life.

There are three factors you need to make a permanent change. The first is a new truth. In this book you'll find the latest information and understanding, expressed simply and unflinchingly – a new truth that you won't find in the mainstream media. The second part of change is emotion, including love, excitement and anger. The love comes from knowing that this is not about deprivation, but about eating again. The excitement comes about when you realise how easy it is and how good you will feel by changing simple habits. The anger comes as you read how the food industry is based on a big fat lie, and when you learn that the foods put on our supermarket shelves are not what they seem. The last part of permanent change is behavioural change. This part is easy, because the new truth and emotion motivate and inspire the change in behaviour.

An unhealthy lifestyle is merely a series of unhealthy habits. To adopt a healthy lifestyle you need to change those habits. I'll show you how to change those unhealthy habits, step by step. Each chapter gives you something to think about and something to act on. Most diets expect you to change everything overnight. That's why most people only stick to such a diet for two to six weeks, and then go back to their old ways. The way to use this book is to read a chapter and then make a change. Each habit change is relatively easy if done by itself. Once you've mastered that single change of habit and it becomes a part of your life, go on to the next change. Changing each bad habit into a good healthy habit might take a week, or it might take longer. It is better to take your time and make sure you've really changed that habit for life. See how much better it makes you feel. This approach can be applied to any unhealthy habits you wish to rid yourself of, such as smoking or drinking. It can also be used in other parts of your life. Every change of habit should be a process of small, achievable steps. Make them a part of your life, then move on. Persistence is the key.

We live in a society that wants quick fixes for everything: 'Get Rich Quick', 'Lose Weight in 10 Days', 'Instant Pain

Relief' and so on. Very few things in life that are achieved quickly are appreciated or maintained. So start making those small, achievable, permanent steps and by the time you have made the final change, you'll feel so very different, bursting with health and energy. Make the commitment now: change one habit per week and don't entertain any other possibility but success. It's worth it.

1

THE BEST WAY
TO START YOUR DAY

*In the past we did what we knew, but now that we know
more, we can do better.*

Breakfast is the perfect place to start your healthy living
program. If you regularly eat breakfast – great! If not, now
is the time to start. But don't just eat anything. If you want to
kick-start your day and have plenty of energy all day long, you
need to eat the right kinds of foods.

The breakfast habit is not an easy one to change, as it's an
embedded part of your morning routine. The tradition seems
to be cereal, toast and tea or coffee. It's only in the western
world where we're cajoled by advertising that we think it perfectly normal to eat rubbish from a box, or the cardboard we
know as toast. Other nations enjoy a healthier start to their
days.

I mean, do you really believe that a box of cereal will make you an iron man? Or that every mouthful is as exciting as a bungee jump? Get real. We are fools to eat devitalised, packaged breakfast cereals. I really believe that eating the cardboard box might be a better option!

To show you how changing your breakfast can change your life, here's a story about a friend of mine. From the age of fifteen she had suffered from dermatitis, arthritis and asthma. At thirty, she was desperate, especially due to her arthritic pain.

I suggested that she change one part of her diet – breakfast. I told her that from the time she woke up until midday the only thing she should eat was fresh fruit, and all she should drink was water. Her normal breakfast was cereal with milk and sugar, toast with margarine and vegemite, and a cup of tea with milk. She would then have another tea with milk every hour or so.

She changed her breakfast habit. The effect was immediate. Within two days the pain she had been experiencing for fifteen years was gone. After a couple of weeks we made more adjustments to her diet following the themes of this book. Within eighteen months she had reduced her use of Ventolin asthma treatment, her dermatitis had disappeared, and there was no arthritic pain. A side benefit was that she went from size 16 to size 8. She incorporated exercise into her life, beginning with a walk five times a week. Twelve years later, she still exercises regularly, works out at the gym three times a week, maintains her changes of habit and remains a size 8. She looks and feels fantastic.

Amazing, isn't it? This all started with one step – changing breakfast. Fruit for breakfast does work for many people, but not all. I'll give you a few more suggestions for a healthy breakfast at the end of this chapter. Choose one of the recipes and stick to it for two weeks.

In winter I like the New Age Porridge, or the Meal on Toast. During summer I enjoy a fruit-only breakfast, the Protein Shake, or Bircher's Muesli. Fruit is a great way to kick-start your day – just keep the fruit bowl handy all morning. The muesli or porridge will sustain you right through to lunchtime, and if it doesn't then have fruit for morning tea.

The Meal on Toast looks pretty easy, but bear in mind that you can't use just any old bread. It needs to be healthy bread. Ezekiel bread (also known as biblical bread) contains wheat, barley, beans, lentils, millet and spelt. The mixture of these legumes and grains creates a complement of amino acids to make a complete protein and a very sustainable bread. Most commercial breads around these days would not sustain life. They're full of additives with very little nutrient value.

The trick is to find a good baker who doesn't use premixes and uses good quality yeast and only the best quality ingredients so you know what's going into the bread you eat. Or buy a bread maker and do it yourself. I recommend a bread maker because then you know exactly what's in the bread you eat. But *do not* use the packet bread mixes! Most packet mixes contain additives and don't have the nutritional value of Ezekiel bread. Make your own bread mix using the recipe on the following page. Make sure you choose organic unbleached flour (available at most grocery stores) and make up the Super Mix – then making your own nutritional bread is a two minute process.

Buying a bread maker is a bit of an outlay, but it is well

worth it. I've noticed that when bread makers first came out, many people bought them, used them once or twice, and then gave them away or sold them to second-hand stores. I picked up my last bread maker in a second-hand shop for a very small amount, and it looked brand-new. If you don't want to buy one or make your own bread, then really question your bakers about what kind of flour and mixes they use. Buy sustainable bread. You'll taste and feel the difference.

Cyndi's Bread

2 cups flour (organic, unbleached plain)
1 cup Super Mix (see below)
1 tbsp cold-pressed oil (macadamia or olive)
1 tsp sea salt
1½ cups water
1 tsp dry yeast or 2cm square of compressed yeast

Mix all ingredients together in a bread maker and press start. For a lighter bread, reduce the Super Mix and replace with organic, unbleached flour.

Super Mix

2 cups rapadura or raw organic sugar
1 cup quinoa or amaranth flour
1 cup sesame seeds
1 cup linseed
1 cup sunflower seeds
1 cup pumpkin seeds
1 cup ground almonds

2 cups organic rolled oats

1 cup maize/polenta

1 cup besan (chickpea) flour

Mix thoroughly and use in bread recipe. Super Mix makes a large batch to save busy people time, but you can make enough for one loaf of bread very easily by substituting each cup measure for a tablespoon measure. You may also need to change amounts according to the size of your bread maker. For a lighter bread leave out the seeds. If you find your bread is a bit heavy, then decrease the Super Mix and replace with plain, organic unbleached flour. Super Mix is a complete protein and can be used for breakfast, with soups, or to make sandwiches.

Breakfast 1 – Protein Shake

1 raw organic free-range egg

1 cup fresh orange juice (or any freshly squeezed juice)

2 tbsp rolled oats

1 tbsp almonds

2 bananas or any fruit you desire

½ cup yoghurt

1 tbsp honey

1 tbsp colloidal minerals (liquid minerals)

1 tbsp cold-pressed oil (macadamia, avocado, flax)

Place in vitamiser and mix. Have with a piece of energy-giving toast, or by itself. This is a complete breakfast, packed with macronutrients (carbohydrates, protein and fats), as well as micronutrients (minerals, vitamins and phytonutrients). The perfect breakfast.

Breakfast 2 – Fruit Only

Have as many pieces of fresh fruit as you want throughout the morning. Have lunch at about midday. With natural foods the body will tell you how much is enough, so don't limit yourself to just a few pieces. You can also make fresh fruit and vegetable juices and have these throughout the morning.

Breakfast 3 – Roasted Kongi

1 cup brown rice
8 cups boiling, filtered water
1 tsp sea salt
1 strip of seaweed (especially for iodine and other minerals) – remove after boiling

Heat a heavy-based frypan over medium–high heat. Add rice and roast until dark brown in colour, stirring constantly so the rice doesn't burn. Put the rice in a saucepan and add boiling water, sea salt and seaweed. Cook covered over low heat until all the water is absorbed – about two hours.

This is a wonderful warm meal but it can also be eaten cold. Keep leftovers in a container in the fridge. The roasting and boiling make the vitamins and minerals in the rice easier to absorb and assimilate.

Eat the roasted kongi with a mix of nuts, seeds, fruit, yoghurt and real maple syrup or honey.

Breakfast 4 – New Age Porridge

1 cup oats

2 cups water

½ tsp sea salt

2 tbsp currants

2 grated apples

1 chopped banana – Cavendish

Mix all ingredients in a saucepan and cook on low heat for about 15 minutes. Serve with maple syrup or honey, or roasted seeds and yoghurt.

Breakfast 5 – Cyndi's Muesli

1 cup rolled oats

2 tbsp sultanas

½ cup orange juice

¼ cup freshly ground nuts

1 grated apple

1 chopped orange

1 mashed banana

½ cup plain yoghurt

2 tbsp natural maple syrup or honey

2 tbsp coconut

Soak oats and sultanas in orange juice overnight. In the morning, add all the other ingredients and mix. You can vary the taste of this cereal by using different fruits, grains, nuts, juices and dried fruits. Try your own variation!

Breakfast 6 – Sweet Meal on Toast
Fresh homemade bread, toasted
Honey
1 mashed banana
Sesame seeds
Pine nuts

Spread honey on the toast, then banana, sesame seeds and pine nuts. Serve with fresh orange juice. Delicious – and full of protein!

Breakfast 7 – Savoury Meal on Toast
Fresh homemade bread, toasted
1 avocado
1 tomato, sliced
Sea salt

Spread avocado on the toast, add the sliced tomato and sprinkle with sea salt – enjoy!

The idea behind these breakfast changes is that you start eating live foods, not dead. By doing this you then become alive with more energy and vitality. That is why fresh fruit is a big part of each breakfast suggestion and why the standard western breakfast habit has to go. Just this one step can make a big difference to the way you feel, the energy you have, and be the beginning of a new way of eating.

ACTION STEPS FOR THIS WEEK

1

Choose one of the breakfast suggestions and stick to it for at least two weeks.

2

If you have children, slowly introduce fruit into their morning routine.

3

Enjoy the increase in energy that you will feel.

2

KEEP CUPPAS
TO A MINIMUM

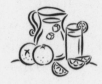

*There is no such thing as a disease that couldn't be
cured. It is people who cannot be cured.*

This week's habit will be a difficult one for some of you to
conquer. But once you've done it, watch out – you'll be
jumping out of your skin with energy!

Are you having trouble sleeping? Feeling nervous, irritable,
agitated, moody, or a bit depressed? Chances are you may be
suffering from an excess of caffeine.

It starts off as a social cuppa. Then it becomes a habit, and
eventually an addiction. Some scientists consider caffeine to be
a powerful and addictive drug because it's very easy to build up
a tolerance. If you drink two cups of coffee a day to get your
caffeine fix this week, then it will probably take three cups a
day to get the same hit next week.

So are you a caffeine addict? An addict is someone who has become dependent on something – tobacco, alcohol, prescription drugs, or caffeine. If you can't get by without your regular cuppa, you are probably addicted. Without that regular hit of caffeine, you would lack concentration, and feel both mentally and physically tired. These are some of the withdrawal symptoms.

Drinking tea or coffee on a regular basis has an effect on every major system in your body. The nervous system suffers the most, as caffeine is a stimulant that affects you mentally and physically. Your bloodstream is also altered, with an increased heart rate and a rise in blood cholesterol and fats which can cause long-term health problems. There is evidence that caffeine can damage your digestive system, increasing the risk of ulcers or aggravating existing ulcers within the stomach. Further down your digestive tract, caffeine-based drinks can reduce the amount of digestive juices in your system, making it more difficult for your body to digest food and reducing the uptake of vital minerals and vitamins you need to produce energy. Large amounts of caffeine (the amount found in six cups of coffee, or two caffeine-enhanced cold drinks, per day) have been linked to high blood pressure and raised cholesterol levels.

Coffee and tea can also affect your kidneys. They act as diuretics, increasing urine flow and causing the loss of important minerals such as calcium, magnesium, sodium and potassium. The additional water loss can even lead to dehydration.

So if caffeine is so bad for us, why not just drink decaffeinated coffee, or tannin-free tea? Well, caffeine is not the only harmful chemical in your favourite cuppa. Teabags contain dyes used to bring out the colour of the tea more quickly, and instant coffee is made using chemicals. These are present in decaffeinated tea and coffee too, so you're no better off for drinking them. And remember, many leading soft drinks, such as cola and the new generation of energy drinks, also contain excessive amounts of caffeine. So make sure you read the labels to check.

It amazes me that probably only 10 per cent of the population has their tea or coffee black. I assume by this that milk or sugar are added to tea and coffee to improve the taste. In other words 90 per cent of people don't really like the taste of tea and coffee so they have to add things to make the drink palatable. Well, why drink the stuff, especially considering it is not that good for you? I believe the experience of having a cuppa is what people actually enjoy, not the drink itself.

Giving up tea or coffee doesn't mean you have to give up the social experience with your hot drinks. In most supermarkets and health food stores you'll find an array of healthy alternatives such as herbal teas. Try them – you'll find one you like. Personally, I love hot water with lemon slices. It's a very refreshing drink, and great for cleaning out the blood and digestive system. I also enjoy most herbal teas but always with lemon slices added. It just seems to give the tea a really uplifting taste. Also try herbal blends (a number of herbs mixed into one tea). I like to go to speciality tea and coffee shops where you can try and then buy.

Of late, chai tea seems to have become a popular drink. This is a mix of black tea with mainly spices. The taste appeals to many people, but chai does contain caffeine. As an alternative you might like to try an amazing tea called Indian spice tea, which is a mix of ginger root, chicory root, carob pod, cardamom seed, cinnamon bark, cinnamon oil, ginger oil, clove bud, stevia leaf and black pepper. It has no black tea and no caffeine and is one of the most refreshing hot drinks I've discovered.

Beware the coffee shop. Powder forms of many hot drinks have taken over from the traditional drinks, and the milk that is used is modified and not in its original or whole form. To have these drinks occasionally is okay, but to drink them on a daily basis is not good for your health. On occasion, I have come across coffee shops that are serving cappuccinos and the like with organic, pasteurised-only milk. Let's hope the trend catches on.

For those of you who are ready to quit the caffeine habit, a word of warning. Cutting down will bring on withdrawal symptoms, including headaches, fatigue, muscle pain or stiffness, and even some flu-like symptoms as your addicted systems cry out for more of the drug. But if you hang in there the symptoms will pass in two or three days and you'll be free of the addiction.

By the way, coffee and tea can be good for you, if drunk the right way. Firstly in moderation and secondly in their natural whole form. Moderation means occasionally. I drink coffee when I need it. If I am speaking out of town and have to drive home late, I will have a coffee around 5.00 p.m., so that my brain stays alert until I get home. If you are not a coffee addict you can safely bet the coffee will keep you alert for up to six hours and sometimes beyond. So I'm usually right until about 11.00 p.m. Used sensibly, coffee can be a great tool for activating the brain for thinking sessions. And I've even heard people say that a cup of good coffee helps take a headache and even a migraine away. This is due to the powerful vasodilator action of the caffeine.

Now for the only coffee or tea you should drink. Whole! That's right – the coffee bean ground and plunged or percolated. The same for tea – whole and in the pot. These then have some health-giving properties in them. But don't spoil them by adding milk and sugar as this has been shown to inhibit the antioxidant properties present in both good tea and coffee.

So drink something different! Change a habit that could be damaging your health into one that is beneficial. Try it – I promise you'll feel better.

ACTION STEPS FOR THIS WEEK

1

Cut out or cut down your coffee and tea habit.

2

Go out and buy some organic lemons and herbal teas.

3

Throw away the instant coffee and tea.

3

DOING THE
CHEWING

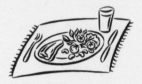

*Without proper digestion there can be no such thing as
good nutrition and health.*

You have to admit that our lives run at a pretty hectic pace,
and it's getting even faster. Food is usually something we
grab on the run and shovel down our throats as quickly as
possible. An exception to this is when we go out for a leisurely
meal – but who has time for that these days?

Sometimes, we don't even have time to chew our food
properly. But I'm here to tell you that it's important to make
the time to eat correctly. If you don't take the time now for
proper digestion, then later in life you will utilise that time
dealing with an array of digestive problems.

To help you understand the importance of this habit, I'll
give you the lowdown on chewing. It plays an important role in

digestion. It's the first step in a long series of events which provide your body with nutrition and energy. If that first step isn't done properly, the entire process can break down. Chewing is the only physical part of the digestive process – the other steps are chemical – so chewing is the only element of digestion that you have total control over. It's great to have control, so use it!

When we chew food properly, two things happen. First, the teeth break the food down into tiny pieces. This increases the surface area of the food, allowing the digestive juices in the stomach to work quickly and effectively. Secondly, the saliva produced in our mouths helps to soften the food and break it down – the first step in a long line of chemical processes.

The more work your mouth does, the less energy you'll need to use for chemical digestion in your stomach and intestines. Chew properly and you'll have less indigestion, burping and flatulence than you've ever had in your life. The more chewing effort you put in, the more physical energy you will have. In short, if you want to be healthy, you need to chew your food well.

Over the years, we've slipped into the habit of bolting our food down quickly. Eating slowly can also become a habit. It's not necessary to count the amount of times you chew each mouthful, just concentrate on chewing your food well.

I've read that repeating an action twenty-one times will turn that action into a habit. Perfect! Three meals a day for seven days gives you twenty-one chances to learn this important new habit. Remembering to do it is the hardest part, so here are a few handy hints. Make your own cue cards or photocopy the following page then cut out the small cards and place them strategically in eating areas where you'll see them. They act as physical reminders to chew your food well. Get the whole family involved and ask them to remind you. Another idea is to have a small cue card in your wallet. When you open it up to buy a meal, you'll see the card and remember.

Slow down your eating. Chew your food well. You'll be investing a few minutes more on your health, but you'll avoid many long hours in the gastroenterologist's waiting room.

ACTION STEPS FOR THIS WEEK

1

Make your own cue cards or photocopy and cut out the cue cards, overleaf.

2

Strategically place them for viewing wherever you eat.

3

Chew more.

CHEW FOOD WELL	CHEW FOOD WELL
SLOW DOWN YOUR EATING	SLOW DOWN YOUR EATING
TAKE TIME TO EAT	TAKE TIME TO EAT
EAT SLOWLY FROM NOW	EAT SLOWLY FROM NOW

4

FOUR PIECES OF
FRESH FRUIT A DAY

*God makes all the healthy food and everything
else is junk.*

CASIE O'MEARA (AGED 7)

The old saying goes, 'An apple a day keeps the doctor away'. It's not far from the truth, but it applies to more than just apples. That's why if you are not already eating fruit for breakfast then this first step in changing your eating habits and improving your life is an important one. Eat at least four pieces of fresh fruit every day. If you want more, go for it!

Fruit is such a fantastic food. It's full of fresh water, vitamins, minerals and fibre. It's alive with enzymes to aid digestion and help clean out the body. And fruit tastes great!

But if you think about what you ate during the last week, how much fruit did you actually consume? Without realising it, you may not be getting your daily intake of fruit. It's just as quick and easy as a bowl of cornflakes at breakfast, or that slice of carrot cake for afternoon tea. So I want you to get into the habit of eating fruit regularly, because it's a vital fuel for your body.

If we look back at the diet of primitive man, our ancestors were basically fruitarians. Before we ever chased a wild pig, we were out chasing berries. Fruit was the staple food. As man evolved, our diet became more varied. We learned to add vegetables, grains, and eventually meat and fish. At first we were not great hunters but wonderful scavengers and meat was a prized food. These changes took place over a period of three million years – a sufficient time period for our bodies to adapt to the alterations. But in the last fifty years, our diet has changed incredibly quickly. We went from fresh healthy foods to refined, manufactured, devitalised food with additives, colours and flavourings and comparatively little nutritional value. Our digestive tracts have had no time to adapt to this new fast food culture, which is so evident when you look at the diseases that are now diet-related. It's time to get back to basics and return to the foods our bodies used to thrive on – like fresh fruit.

Fresh fruit is a delicious form of energy. It's packed with fructose (a simple sugar), phytonutrients, fibre, vitamins and minerals. As fruit also has a very high water content, it acts as an excellent body cleanser, flushing out impurities. Plus it can help get rid of waste from your digestive system, bloodstream, internal organs, and even your skin.

When you go to sleep at night, your metabolism and digestive system slow down. A good way to wake your body and kick-start your digestive system is to begin your day with some fruit. It's easy to digest, helps with bowel regularity, and increases the body's metabolic rate.

So what kind of fruit should you eat? The key is variety. Each kind of fruit has different types of vitamins, minerals, amino acids, carbohydrates, fats and water, in different amounts. These days, you can find a huge variety of fruits available all year round, so make the most of it! In my opinion, you can never have too much fresh fruit. Four pieces per day is a guideline. And I don't mean four grapes or cherries – I mean an apple, a banana and an orange or pear, or a large section of rockmelon, watermelon, a bunch of grapes and mandarins. No cheating on this one – you need at least four *serious* pieces of fruit a day.

To help you remember to eat your fruit it is a good idea to have a bowl of fruit on your desk at work, a bowl of fruit on display in your house, and to always grab some fruit when you drive in the car.

It is important to wash your fruit. As soon as I get home from the market I put everything in the sink and give it a good wash. This is to clean off any sprays or residues on the skin.

Buying organic fruit is the best option, and more and more people are demanding this produce so the availability and price are becoming more competitive. The great thing about organic fruit is that it is free from chemical sprays, and what's even better is that organic fruit has a higher vitamin, mineral and nutrient content than the non-organic variety. The principle of organic farming is that a healthy plant grows from good healthy soil and as a result it should be able to resist pests and disease. Therefore the farmer can avoid synthetic fertilizers or chemical pesticides. Organically grown food is produced from natural farming systems that do not damage the environment. The management of organic farming requires more skill and hard work than simply spraying a field with poisons. Therefore the lower cost of conventionally grown food does not represent the true cost of increased health care, environmental clean up and the permanent loss of good topsoil.

The chemicals that have been used and are being used in the production of foods have strong links to many diseases, ailments and discomforts. The chemicals I refer to belong to the family group of organochlorines known as the cyclodienes. These include DDT, dieldrin, aldrin, endrin, heptachlor, isobenzane, lindane and chlordane. These chemicals are particularly persistent in the environment and have been found in human milk. The following is by no means a complete list but symptoms that have been identified as a result of chemical exposure include rashes, sweating, joint and muscle pains, fatigue, lymph node swelling, swollen glands, persistent diarrhoea, allergies, anxiety, twitching eyelids, muscular spasm, heart palpitations, vision blackouts, cancer and death.

It is worth making the effort to find good quality organic food. You'll feel more healthy, energetic and alive with more fruit in the diet – ready for the next good health habit.

ACTION STEPS FOR THIS WEEK

1

Fill the fridge with fruit.

2

Have a bowl of fruit on the office desk.

3

Fill a bag of fruit for the car.

4

Display a bowl of fruit in the house.

5

Search out organic fruit and vegetable suppliers. (See page 261.)

5

WATER –
WHERE TO GET IT

It is better for you to take responsibility for your life as
it is instead of blaming others, or circumstances, for
your predicament.

DAN MILLMAN

Sixty-five to 70 per cent of your body is made up of water.
So if you weigh sixty kilos, around forty kilos of that is
water. Without it, you'd look like a sultana rather than a grape.

So we know we need water, but how much is enough? In a
temperate climate, the estimate is about three litres per day.
Consuming that much water can be hard work, especially if it's
ghastly town water. But there are other ways to get the water
you need.

Did you know that fresh fruits and vegetables contain anywhere between 60 and 90 per cent water? It's good water too,

so eating plenty of fresh fruit and vegies will reduce your need to guzzle litres of the wet stuff every day. It's not just fruit and vegies either – you'll find a high water content in sprouted seeds and legumes plus cooked grains including oatmeal, rice and barley, and cooked legumes such as lentils, red kidney beans and chickpeas.

There's another important point I'd like to talk about now – the difference between liquids and water. Let's use coffee as an example. Yes coffee contains water, but that doesn't mean your body is able to retain the water and use it.

As we have already discussed, tea and coffee both contain substances which can cause the body to lose water, upsetting the water balance of your body. Soft drinks, fruit juices and cordials, which are high in sugar, can also contribute to the change in osmotic pressure of a cell. And of course alcohol (like tea and coffee) is a diuretic, causing you to lose water by going to the toilet more than usual. That's why you end up with a hangover after drinking – because your body and brain are dehydrated. The things we do to our bodies in the name of fun!

Many people ask me if they should drink fluids with their meals. To me, there is no black and white answer to this. A lot of alternative health professionals advise that you should not drink water with meals because it dilutes the digestive juices. In my opinion, it depends on the content of the meal. Saliva is 99 per cent water, which suggests that we need water to digest our food.

Let's take a look at two breakfasts. The first is a dry cereal with a small amount of milk and sugar, and toast with butter and honey. The second is a piece of fresh fruit, then oatmeal, grated apple, yogurt and honey. Compare the two. The first has virtually no water content, but the second breakfast is swimming in it. Eat the first meal and your body will signal it needs water, but with the second meal, the need for fluids will be little or nothing, because the water is within the meal.

So if you eat a dry or salty meal then by all means follow your body's instincts and drink water. But try a meal of fruit, vegies or salads and find out how great water tastes when it's packaged by Mother Nature.

The water that comes out of our taps is not like the fresh clean water of a mountain stream or the filtered water within organic fruits and vegetables. The water from the tap usually has many additives. The additives come from many sources, from the council who add chlorine and fluoride, to the dangerous chemicals from farms where there is a runoff into our dams. Recycled waste can also be in the water supply, and the list goes on. To get rid of most of these additives, get yourself a water filter. Even though it requires some capital outlay, they are well worth it. I would rather have a water filter doing most of the work than allowing my kidneys and the rest of my body to do it. Wear out the water filter, not your body. Make sure you use this filtered water in cooking as well as drinking.

An even smarter idea, in these days of expensive water rates and restrictions, is to attach a water tank to the house.

I recommend that at least 70 per cent of your diet should be water based, because after all our brain and body are 65 to 70 per cent water. This is easy to do. Just make sure your diet consists of more high water content foods such as fruits, vegies, salads, rice, soups, sprouts, cooked legumes and glasses of filtered water.

ACTION STEPS FOR THIS WEEK

1

Write out your diet for a day and see how much of it is water based.

2

Look around for a good water filter.

3

See if your local council will subsidise a water tank.

4

Eat a diet that is at least 70 per cent water based.

6

QUALITY VS QUANTITY

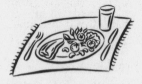

It is a miracle that curiosity survives a formal education.
ALBERT EINSTEIN

'Insanity is doing the same thing and expecting a different result' – one of my favourite sayings. In other words, if you continue to do what you are doing right now then you will continue to get the same results. Change what you are doing and a new result will follow. I know this sounds like commonsense, but I'm finding that commonsense is no longer that common.

I get many phone calls, questions and emails asking if I can help people with their diet as far as it relates to diabetes. It seems there is no other disease out there that is affecting such a vast number of the population. In fact, in the last 20 years the incidence of diabetes has increased a whopping 300 per cent.

I hear of young fit men and women competing in triathlons

and marathons – competitors who are fit and, we would assume, healthy – dying of heart attacks. And these are not old people – these are people in their twenties and thirties.

Cancer rates are escalating, and they now say that everyone in Australia will be affected in some way by it, whether by association or by having cancer themselves. The way the statistics are going, by the year 2020 every male in the western world will have cancer.

If you go to your Internet search engine and type in 'diseases starting with A', you will be astounded at how many diseases begin with that letter – then make your way through the alphabet. There seems to be more diseases than the population of a medium-sized town.

The latest craze in printing on T-shirts for obese children is, 'The fat kid always wins at see-saw'. This tells me that there are enough obese or overweight people out there who will buy the T-shirt to make the manufacturers some money. It's become a joke rather then a serious health problem.

Hold the bus! What is happening out there? Thirty years ago we were pretty healthy and average in weight compared to what we are now. What's the difference?

Over the past 30 years the diet industry and many health professionals have pushed the low-fat, low-calorie, high-carbohydrate diet for weight control and disease control. And in the last 30 years our health has hit an all-time low and our weight has hit an all-time high. The main theme of every diet book, whether it is for weight loss or health, is to look at how much of each food group you eat, how many calories, how many grams, how much fat, how big a plate, smaller portion sizes, etc. If you haven't figured it out by now, this book takes the focus away from the amount of food you should be eating and concentrates on the *quality* of the food you eat, and what's amazing is that when you begin to concentrate on the quality of the food, then the quantity issue sorts itself out.

Thirty years ago food was less about technology and more about nature; there were fewer chemicals and more vitamins and minerals, and less part-foods and more wholefoods. Now we eat mainly technology-driven foods rather then nature-based foods, and that is where we are failing.

To me it is a no-brainer! Eat well and you will be healthy. Concentrate on quality and less on quantity. Now I can hear you all saying, but what is eating well? What is a healthy food or quality food? One day we are told something is good for us and then the next day it causes one of the new diseases of the alphabet, or cancer. So everyone throws up their hands in horror and says they'll eat what they want.

Well, guess what? This book is about eating what you want: chocolate cake, ice-cream, cappuccino, chips, bacon and eggs, butter, and so on. What is more important then anything else is the *quality* of the ingredients that make up these foods. It makes all the difference.

It's time to stop thinking so hard about 'how much' and to start thinking more about 'how good'. If the quality is top-notch, then the body will be able to tell you intuitively about the quantity. But we also have to use some commonsense here. Although organic butter is a quality food, you wouldn't eat nothing but butter for your nutrition. An array of quality foods from all the food groups is the answer.

The body is extraordinary – if you have the right amount of vitamins and minerals, then it has a mechanism by which it will not crave foods and will achieve satiety.

A craving is merely the body saying 'you don't have enough vitamins and minerals, eat more food'. But instead of eating vitamin- and mineral-packed food, as we would have done just 30 short years ago, we now eat chocolate, chips and snack foods, and therefore we don't give the body what it needs. So it asks for more. The vicious cycle begins and we eat vast quantities of wasted calorie food, instead of eating *good quality* vitamin- and mineral-rich food, resulting in obesity and major health problems.

Most foods can be healthy – it all depends on the quality of the ingredients. Even chocolate cake can be healthy. Let's compare a healthy chocolate cake to a chocolate cake that should be avoided at all costs.

Healthy Chocolate Cake	Chocolate Cake to Be Avoided
Ingredients	Ingredients
· Organic, unbleached flour	· Baker's flour
· Organic rapadura sugar	· White or artificial sugar
· Butter	· Margarine or hydrogenated vegetable oil
· Organic cocoa, without colours or flavourings	· Cocoa flavouring
· Organic free-range eggs	· Egg substitute
· Pasteurised-only milk	· Skim milk powder and water
	· Brown colouring, additives, preservatives and flavourings

Can you see the difference? Some people cook with ingredients from the right-hand side, and most bought cakes are made with these and even more additives. Why not make a chocolate cake with the best ingredients? Taste the difference and feel the difference. When you eat the Chocolate Cake to be Avoided you often don't feel good after it, but when you eat the Healthy Chocolate Cake you won't have the same sick feeling.

Looking at all your foods, and the ingredients of all the foods you prepare, and making sure the quality is there will begin to improve health. The ultimate in quality foods are freshly picked organic produce; freshly milled organic grains; organic nuts freshly cracked; dairy straight from an organically fed cow; oils that have been cold pressed using organic ingredients; organic meat, chicken and fish from non-polluted waters; and the dream goes on. While these are the ultimate, they are often not practical in our western lives. So okay, we can't do the best, but we can get pretty close. It is just a matter of educating yourself about what is out there and taking steps to improve quality.

Taking a step-by-step approach to changing the quality of food is the easiest way to go. Begin with the pantry: when you use up a particular food, seek its highest quality version to replace it. For instance, change to organic, unbleached flour. Go from white salt to sea salt (it's moist but it has a greater amount of nutrients). When the white sugar runs out, try rapadura, sucanat or muscovado (dehydrated sugarcane juice). Tins of tomatoes, chickpeas, tuna and corn can be replaced with tinned organic varieties. If you buy pasta sauces, choose organic ones. Change your white pasta to organic pasta, or pasta made from quinoa or another grain. Food by food, you can change to better quality products. Most of these foods can be found in the supermarket at a similar price.

All your nuts, seeds and legumes should be fresh, without any additives. Cheese, butter, milk, cream and sour cream are now available organic and in their purest form. Pasteurised-only milk is the best you can buy and organic is readily available in the supermarket. When it comes to yoghurt, the old-fashioned yoghurt without any additives can't be beaten. For juices, check that they are pure juice with very few additives and preservatives. The best choice, of course, is to drink freshly squeezed juice, and with the proliferation of juice bars that isn't hard to do any more.

Meat and chicken should be organic. These are concentrated foods that store unwanted chemicals that are not really good for human health.

Organic is always best, of course, but even having fresh fruit and vegetables in your fridge is a bonus. I've been to some people's homes where there are neither fruit nor vegetables in sight – maybe the canned and frozen variety, but nothing fresh.

Throughout the book, the benefits of all these wonderful foods will be explained.

You are what you eat. Eat quality foods and you will have a quality body. How can you possibly think that your muscle, blood vessels and other body structures can be at peak performance unless you have the right building blocks? It's time to put more thought into quality and less into quantity.

ACTION STEPS FOR THIS WEEK

1

Start becoming aware of how often you think in terms of how much you can have.

2

Look at the quality of the food you're eating, taking particular notice of the ingredients.

3

Read all food labels (the next chapter will help you understand them).

7

HEALTHY READING

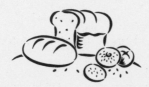

*Your thoughts create a direct physical effect on
your body.*

I will consistently tell you to read all food labels. But reading
food labels is a bit like looking into a crystal ball. It's all
guesswork, unless you know what you're looking for.

This week's habit is all about improving your knowledge of
the processed foods you are eating. This should allow you to
make informed choices about the foods you buy and eat.

Let's start at the beginning, where farmers grow the basic
ingredients: fruits, vegetables and grains. These crops are often
grown under less than favourable conditions with artificial fertilisers and chemical pesticides. Then, after picking, some of
the foods are preserved using chemical powders and sprays.

But wait a minute! None of that appears on the packaging!

That's because they don't have to tell you what happens to your food *before* it gets to the manufacturer or cannery. And if that gets your blood boiling, that's just the tip of the iceberg!

Australian law says that all packaged and tinned foods must have the ingredients listed on the packaging. Those ingredients must be listed in descending order of weight. Here's an example for you: 'Sugar, glucose syrup, plums, vegetable gum (415), food acid (330), colour (128)'. Can you guess what food that makes up? Believe it or not, it's jam. According to my old grandma's recipe, jam was supposed to be made from equal parts fruit and sugar, and pectin. But in the above jam, there's more sugar than there is fruit plus other things that perhaps you would be better off not eating.

Often when people look at food labels they don't seem to look at the ingredients, but rather at the percentage of fat, carbohydrates and proteins. In my way of thinking, this portion of the label is the last thing to look at. The most important thing to read is the ingredients. You want to make sure that the food you are eating is from nature and not from technology. Remember, the issue here is the quality of the food not the quantity and percentage of the macronutrients (carbohydrates, protein and fat). Once you have established that the quality of the food in the package is natural, then you can have a look at the other information. For example, you may have a very low-fat food but the ingredients may all be of very low quality, whereas another food label may have a higher fat content but the quality of the food is far superior. See the two labels following.

Nutrition Facts

Serving Size: ½ Pack (5 oz/142.5g)
Servings Per Pack: 2

	Quantity per serve	Quantity per 100g
Energy	138Kcal	96.6Kcal
Protein	4.3g	3g
Total fat	9.6g	6.7g
Saturated Fat	2g	1.4g
Carbohydrates		
Total	8.6g	6g
Sugars	2.1g	1.5g
Dietary Fibre	4g	2.8g
Cholestrol	2.6mg	1.8mg
Sodium	416.5mg	291.6mg

INGREDIENTS: GREEN PEAS (31%), SPINACH (3.6%),
TOMATOES, ONIONS, FENUGREEK, CASHEW NUTS,
CREAM, WATERMELON SEEDS, SUNFLOWER OIL,
SALT, GARLIC, GINGER, HERBS & SPICES, WATER

This is a packaged food found on many grocery shelves. If you look at the ingredients, it is something that you would make at home. There are no artificial additives or unusual ingredients. But when you go to the percentage of fat, carbohydrates and protein, you may think it is not a good food because it contains 11.6 grams of fat per serving, including 2 grams of saturated fat. And if you live by the old rules, where fat – especially saturated fat – is a no-no, then you may put this package down and look for something with less fat.

Let's compare it to another shelf item with far less fat.

INGREDIENTS: JELLY (WATER, SUGAR, FOOD ACIDS (327, 330, 331), VEGETABLE GUMS (410, 415, 418), COLOURS (VEGETABLE YELLOW, 133), LIME FLAVOUR, ANTIOXIDANT (ASCORBIC ACID)) (72%), PEAR (28%)

NUTRITION INFORMATION

SERVES PER PACK: 4		SERVING SIZE: 120g
AVERAGE QUANTITY	PER SERVE	PER 100g
ENERGY	372KJ	310KJ
PROTEIN	0.2g	0.2g
FAT-TOTAL	0.1g	0.1g
-SATURATED	NIL	NIL
CARBOHYDRATE	22.8g	19.0g
-SUGARS	21.6g	18.0g
DIETARY FIBRE	1.1g	0.9g
SODIUM	60mg	50mg

This food has only 0.1 gram of fat, and no saturated fat, but its ingredients are totally artificial. So if you only look at the percentages of the macronutrients and you fail to look at the ingredients, you are missing the true picture.

Another little trick that you may need to know: you'll see on the food labels that nutritional content is expressed in grams rather than as a percentage of the ingredients. In this way the consumer can be tricked into believing that something is low in fat, when in fact the fat content might be quite high. Fat has 9 calories per gram, and protein and carbohydrates are 4 calories per gram – a percentage figure would provide a more accurate, and off-putting, picture. But remember that the most important thing is the quality of the fat you are eating (more on that later, in the chapter on fat).

Your next step on the journey to decipher food labels are those interesting numbers in brackets. Since January 1987, food companies have been required to identify the additives they use, rather than using vague terms like colouring or preservative. But unless you know how to decode those numbers, you still don't know what you're eating.

I recommend that you buy *Additive Alert* by Julie Eady or *The Chemical Maze* by Bill Statham. These books give you plenty of detail on all the numbers, including their names, their function, what foods the additives are used in, and any known harmful effects. Some of these additives are harmless substances which help to keep processed food safe to eat, yet there are others which are inessential, and can be harmful to some people.

Basically the numbering system works like this: numbers between 100 and 180 are colours; 200 to 290 are preservatives; 300 to 320 are antioxidants; 322 to 494 are emulsifiers; and numbers 905 to 907 are mineral hydrocarbons.

The use of colourings is a debatable issue when discussing food additives. Colourings are purely cosmetic and serve no particular purpose for the preservation and taste of foods. The Hyperactive Children's Support Group has recommended the avoidance of the following numbers: 102, 107, 110, 120, 122, 123, 124, 127, 132, 133, 150, 151, 155, 160b, 210, 211, 220, 250, 251, 319, 320, 321, 421, 620, 621, 627, 631, 635 and 951. Notice that the majority are colours and are usually found in children's treats.

Specifically, 621 – a flavour enhancer known as Monosodium Glutamate, or MSG, and often disguised as hydrolysed vegetable protein – is an additive to avoid. Current research is implicating it as contributing to the obesity epidemic. One reason is that it addicts people to the food it is put in – you can't eat just one. It is not permitted in food for babies due to its effect on the central nervous system. Other adverse reactions to this additive are depression, mood changes, sleeplessness, nausea, migraine, abdominal discomfort and convulsions. Read the labels and try to avoid it as much as possible.

The following additives can be dangerous for asthmatics and people sensitive to aspirin. They should also be avoided by hyperactive children and adults, and should not be permitted in food for babies and young children. They are: 212, 213, 216, 218, 221–224, 310–312, 621–623, 627 and 631. Possible carcinogenic (cancer forming) additives are: 110, 123, 131, 142, 210, 211, 213, 214–217, 239, 249–252, 330, 321, 407, 431–433, 435, 436, 466, 530, 553, 900, 914, 943a, 950–952, 954, 967 and 1201. These lists are by no means complete. I recommend you buy Julie's book and get a complete list of additives to avoid.

Most additives do serve a purpose in the processed food industry, but it is whether we choose to eat a diet full of processed food that decides how many of these additives we are exposed to. Choosing a diet of whole natural foods will ensure that your exposure to any dangerous additives is minimal.

There is another factor to be aware of when you read food labels. Let's say a food producer buys an ingredient such as glucose from another company. That glucose may contain additives, such as sulphur dioxide (220), but the purchasing food producer doesn't have to acknowledge that. All they have to mention on the label is glucose syrup. Current legislation allows for food manufacturers not to declare components of ingredients that make up less than 5 per cent of a product, and as a result there are many products on the market that contain additives that are not declared on the label. Become informed so that you know what you are eating.

And that's just the start. That magic word – added – has a hidden agenda. If you see the words 'no added sugar' it actually means that there *is* sugar added, just that the added amount is less than the legal limit needed to put sugar on the ingredients list. Using fruit juice as an example, the manufacturer can add sugar up to 4 per cent of the volume of the drink without having to declare it on the label. Also beware of the word added in front of MSG, salt and other additives as it still means an amount they can legally put in without having to declare it. It can also mean that the food manufacturer has not added it, but it may be in some of the ingredients purchased to make the product.

Another word you'll see frequently on food packaging is 'natural'. You'd think a natural product would be in its whole state and free of any additives. Be careful here! Read the ingredients and you will see that not all the ingredients are natural or in their whole state. For instance, natural yoghurt will usually contain concentrated skim milk. This is not food in its natural state, but rather one that has been through some processing.

This has a further impact. It means that when you read the words 'no artificial flavourings', the product probably contains natural flavourings. But remember, they may come from a natural source but not be in their natural state after processing. Only if the label says 'no flavourings', can you feel confident that it contains none at all.

The use of the word 'organic' is another issue. Make sure when you see 'organic' on a label that you also see a certifying symbol from an authorised agency for their seal of approval – but more on that in the chapter on organics.

It is a maze out there with food labelling. Some additives cause health problems whereas others are thought not to be dangerous. Many additives are said to be totally safe but it is important to remember that they may have been in the food chain for only a short time. They are not wholefoods, but chemicals extracted by manipulating foods and substances. Even though I have given you numbers to avoid, you should be aware of *all* food additives. By educating yourself on the additive and number system you can then become an aware buyer. You can help prevent the use of dangerous additives by choosing goods without suspect substances and choosing carefully where you shop. The consumer can have an influence on the composition and production of foods.

So, there's the lowdown on reading food labels. Next time you go to the supermarket, start reading the labels. You might try one product at a time, or one aisle per shopping trip. It'll take time initially, but eventually you'll work through the shopping list and know which foods and brands are best for your family.

Once you have done this, don't think you can then become complacent. Manufacturers are continually changing their ingredients, probably for cheaper costs and better profits, or a better tasting food or drink. So periodically check the food you have become comfortable with to make sure the ingredients have not changed.

ACTION STEPS FOR THIS WEEK

1

Start by reading food labels in your pantry.

2

Buy *Additive Alert* by Julie Eady
(www.additivealert.com.au), or
The Chemical Maze by Bill Statham
(www.thechemicalmaze.com).

3

Make up a card with all the additives that are
dangerous to your health and carry it on your
trips to the supermarket, or send for a card from
www.changinghabits.com.au.

4

Choose foods that do not harm.

8

FRANKENSTEIN
FOODS

*Genetic engineering of our food has the potential to be
the most damaging thing for the environment and our
health, and the effects will be irreversible.*

To eat or not to eat, that is the question. Genetically modified (GM) foods were sneaked into our food supply as
early as 1996. It is only recently that all hell has broken loose.
Slowly the news leaked out that GM products were in the
foods that we buy. A significant percentage of the population
who had decided they didn't want this made a hullabaloo about
it and, not surprisingly, the concern over these foods is growing.

I telephoned one food company about it. They had been
using GM products in the manufacture of their foods, but they
told me that once their supplies had run out (in about three

months or so) they would source GM-free foods. What concerned me was that this manufacturer makes foods for infants. They should have thought twice before even using these Frankenstein foods.

I look at it this way. If you choose not to be aware of GM foods and the products they are in, then you become part of the biggest uncontrolled experiment of all time, because we are being exposed to these foodstuffs constantly. Nobody knows the results, nobody can tell us if there are long-term effects, and to tell you honestly, I simply will not be a part of such an experiment.

The situation is a bit like the chemicals that have been used to produce our food since the fifties. At the time they were believed to be safe, so everyone sprayed them on our foods with gay abandon. But forty years on, we are seeing the harm that these chemicals can do to our health.

It is also like the fat issue. We have been duped into believing that margarine and polyunsaturated fats (man-made) are better for us than natural fats. The people who choose to eat them have been part of an experiment, the conclusions being that these man-made fats could be one of the major contributors to heart disease, cancer and diabetes. (More on that later.)

With these two major catastrophes how can we possibly believe that GM foods are safe?

So what are genetically modified foods, and why do we need them? The theory is basically to modify the genetic structure of a plant so as to improve on nature, to feed a hungry world, to produce edible vaccines and to produce crops which are resistant to attack by pests and therefore use less chemical spray.

Let's look at each of these aspects.

I cannot believe the audacity of science! We're so arrogant that we think we can improve on nature. Nature has given us everything we need to evolve. We can be healthy humans if we eat the foods we have evolved to consume. Haven't we learnt from past mistakes? Most foods that have been changed by technology, such as margarine, artificial sweeteners and modified milks, have been a disaster for health.

The world is hungry – not for lack of food, but for beliefs, politics and administration. There is so much waste in the western world and in the inefficient production of many foods. Lack of food is not our problem. As Ghandi said, 'This planet will provide for man's needs, not for man's greed'. And I see GM foods as a greed issue. As for edible vaccines, I'm not too happy about the thought of mass medication and full-scale human experimentation.

The statement that GM foods are designed to produce crops resistant to attack by pests or weeds goes beyond my comprehension. The first crop to be engineered were soybeans made resistant to a herbicide, which normally killed them, but now only kills the competing weeds. To me, that does not make a plant resistant to pests, but rather resistant to chemicals, and what is the purpose of that? It comes as no surprise that the chemical companies and the makers of GM foods are linked.

The most frightening aspect about GM foods is what is known as 'terminator technology'. The theory behind this is that the plant is genetically modified so that it will not produce a viable seed to ensure the future of that plant, therefore making it impossible for farmers to save and replant seeds. The consequence of this is that farmers will have to buy the seed each year from the same company. This to me has serious social, economic, health and environmental implications. Thank goodness there are people out there who are saving viable seeds.

I am not one to fool with food or nature, and I believe that GM foods and terminator technology is a dangerous step away from nature.

By decree of Food Standards Australia New Zealand (FSANZ), there should be no genetically modified fresh fruit, vegetables, meat, poultry or fish in the Australian and New Zealand food supply, but there are currently six GM foods and their 19 derivatives (additives, flavourings, flour, etc.) that may be sold: soy, sugar beet, corn, cottonseed oil, canola and potatoes. Since 7 December 2001, labels must inform if a food contains novel genetic material or genetically modified protein introduced by genetic modification. This information will usually be in the ingredients list.

One of the main sources of GM ingredients in food sold in Australia is soy. It is found in biscuits, bread, chocolate, margarine, mayonnaise and potato chips, to name a few. Cottonseed oil produced from GM cotton is used for frying in the food industry and is found in mayonnaise and salad dressings. GM corn can be found in imported foods like breakfast cereals, bread, corn chips and gravy mixes. Some imported foods may have the following GM ingredients: potatoes, canola oil, sugar beet, yeast, cauliflower and coffee.

Consumer demand is a powerful thing, so much so that some food manufacturers in Australia have taken steps to provide GM-free food. These products may be labelled accordingly, by stating 'contains no genetically modified ingredients'. For more information, including a list of foods and brands that are GM-free, contact Greenpeace. Search their website in your area, and become an educated consumer who says no to the manipulation of food and nature.

ACTION STEPS FOR THIS WEEK

1

Search the Internet, or phone Greenpeace for a copy of their GM-free food list.
http://sites.greenpeace.org.au/truefood/guide2.html

2

Look in your pantry and see how GM-free you are.

3

When shopping next, choose only GM-free foods.

9

SALT OF

THE EARTH

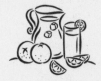

*If you want your life to change then you must
first change.*

How many times have you been told to reduce your salt
intake? If you're eating too much of it, that's fair enough.
But if you're only using a little salt as a condiment, then don't
change the amount you're using – change the *kind* of salt
you're using.

From the day we are conceived until the day that we die, we
need salt. But a lot of people aren't aware that the salt we eat
nowadays is a refined food containing additives. If we ate salt in
its raw state, it would be considered a health food like other
mineral supplements. Every day we are told about the bad
effects of refined foods, and salt is no exception. The table and
cooking salt we use is almost completely devoid of nutrition: it

is a chemical substance which can contribute to oedema, excess weight, high blood pressure, kidney disease, liver congestion and arteriosclerosis.

So what's wrong with refined salt? Well, during the refining process, up to eighty-two trace minerals and essential nutrients are destroyed by the 1200-degree heating process, leaving only one compound – sodium chloride. Without the other minerals to counteract some of its effects, high intake of sodium chloride can cause muscle weakness and can be linked to calcium store depletion. This may be part of the reason why osteoporosis has become so common of late.

But it's not only what the manufacturers take out during the refining process; it's what they put in. Because salt absorbs water from the atmosphere, additives are mixed with it to prevent it from becoming lumpy. The additives are bleaches and anti-caking agents, such as calcium phosphate monabasic (341), sodium aluminosilicate (554), and aluminium calcium silicate (556).

But you don't have to eat refined salt. Take a trip to your nearest health food store or the health food section of your supermarket and pick up some unrefined sea salt. It's not sparkling white like refined salt, but it's a hell of a lot better for you. I use unrefined sea salt in my cooking as well as on the table, although you will have to throw away your salt shaker as the sea salt tends to clog it up. Use a salt pig instead. Salt is most easily digested and assimilated when cooked or in pickled food because it has dissolved and separated into its constituent ions.

I ask many people whether they eat salt and because of the

campaign against salt (due to its connection with hypertension) many have taken it out of their diet completely. Our soils are very depleted of valuable minerals and, as a result, so are the foods that are grown in it. I suggest you put salt back into your diet; but only in moderation and only unrefined sea salt.

I note here that sea salt does not contain iodine, a very important mineral essential for health, and especially needed for the integrity and health of the thyroid. Many soils are deficient in iodine, therefore the food grown in these soils is also deficient. The best sources of iodine are seaweeds such as kelp, nori, wakami and the like. Combining sea salt with finely chopped seaweed will ensure you get an adequate supply of iodine and the other essential minerals for health. If you like Japanese food, especially nori rolls, make them part of your weekly eating regime.

The moral of today's habit is one you'll hear from me again and again – natural is better. I can think of no better way to illustrate this than by sharing the results of an experiment with you. Several years ago a team of eminent scientists analysed some sea-water, then manufactured their own by duplicating the chemical analysis as closely as possible. They set up two tanks filled with plankton – one containing the natural seawater, the other filled with the man-made copy. They then added fish. Although these liquids were chemically identical, twenty-four hours later the fish in the real seawater were thriving, while the fish in the man-made seawater were dead. Like I say, natural is better.

So your task for this week is to go through your pantry and throw out all your refined table and cooking salt. Then head for the health food store and stock up with natural, unrefined sea salt. It can be bought as coarse, medium or fine. What you choose will depend on how you intend to use it. Coarse sea salt is good for soups and vegetables, but the fine sea salt is a far better option for the table and for baking. As a matter of preference, I buy fine granules. This simple step is another towards health, energy and vitality, because every time you eat sea salt, you are actually eating a multi-mineral complex.

ACTION STEPS FOR THIS WEEK

1

Throw away the white refined salt.

2

Go and buy some grey unrefined sea salt.

3

Add finely chopped seaweed to your sea salt for iodine.

4

Start using the multi-mineral health giving sea salt.

10

THE FACTS
ON FAT

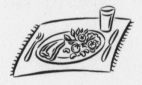

*It's not what happens to us in life but rather how we
handle what happens that matters.*

For the last ten years or so, the food industry has been
pushing the low-fat revolution. But despite our national
obsession to get rid of fat from our diets, a decade down the
track we are even fatter than we were! In fact, nationally, 61
per cent of males, 56 per cent of females and a staggering 30
per cent of children are obese, and the figures are rising. Glob-
ally, 1.5 billion adults and 10 per cent of children are
overweight or obese – it is becoming known as 'globesity'. So
what is going on?

For starters, let's clear up the myth that fat is bad for you.
That is not necessarily the case. Humans need fat to be healthy –
it provides the structure of many cell components. We need fat

to help us manufacture many vital compounds, and to take up fat-soluble vitamins (A, D, E and K) and other nutrients known as carotenoids.

There is so much ignorance about the importance of fat. Australians have been conned by the food industry into believing that low fat means non-fattening and healthy. This is just not true! What the food industry does is take good natural foods and manipulate them into what I term fake foods, all so they can enjoy the marketing benefit and profits of calling them low fat or lite. The truth is that fats are not taboo. Foods containing natural fats will not cause ill health, as long as they are eaten in their natural state and are part of a diet that has lots of fruits, vegetables, grains, nuts, seeds, eggs and meat.

Let's look at the history of fats. For thousands of years humans have eaten a variety of fats, from both animals (saturated) and vegetables (unsaturated). These fats have been needed for the evolution of our brain and nervous system. It is believed that fats were, and still are, important for the evolution and sophistication of the human brain. Both saturated and unsaturated fats are needed for a healthy nervous system, a healthy liver, enhanced immune system, depression of tumour growth, transport of essential fatty acids, hormone production, successful blood clotting and satiety (to signal when you have eaten enough). Really I have only touched the surface by telling you how important both saturated and unsaturated fats are for the body.

Back in the early part of last century the average westerner would get most of their fat from animal sources, and less from polyunsaturated oils and margarine. The fats that were eaten were tallow, lard and butter. Back then, lifestyle diseases such as heart disease and cancer were minimal. In fact cancer affected 3 per cent of the population and myocardial infarction was a minor problem – unlike today, when dietary fats are mainly polyunsaturated from sources such as hydrogenated oils and margarines, while animal fats have become taboo. In the scientific community it is a well-known fact that these technology fats – mainly hydrogenated fats or trans fats – inhibit cell membrane function; decrease hormone production, leading to infertility; interfere with the enzyme systems the body needs to eliminate carcinogens and toxins, which in turn contributes to cancer; and inhibit insulin receptors contributing to the cause of type 2 diabetes. Disastrously, hydrogenated fats in the diet of pregnant women contribute to low birth weight babies and inhibit visual and neurological function, and they lower fat content in mothers' milk, which can depress learning ability, predominantly in situations of stress. Recent research indicates that hydrogenated fats are more likely to cause weight gain than any other fat.

People are paranoid about the word fat and more particularly saturated fat. I would like to change that. And to make you paranoid . . . not about natural fats but about the fats that man has made, and manipulated, and incorporated into most of the foods that we eat, from biscuits to breakfast cereals and most prepared or packaged foods.

Without fats in the diet there are no essential fatty acids. Essential fatty acids are fats that we must eat for health, as our body cannot manufacture them. Recent surveys show that at least 80 per cent of the western population is deficient in the essential fatty acids. This lack of essential fatty acids has been implicated in the increase in multiple sclerosis, cancer, and Attention Deficit Hyperactivity Disorder (ADHD); once again these are just a token of the problems that are showing up as possible results of this deficiency.

Any weight loss diet usually has minimal fats and an increase in carbohydrates. What confuses me is that when animals need fattening all fats in their diet are restricted while the amount of grain and cereals (carbohydrates) is increased. That means when we humans go on a fat free diet we are actually following a fattening – rather than a weight loss – program. Statistics show that 97 per cent of people who go on a fat and calorie restricting diet reduce their weight, but twelve months later are fatter than when they started.

Have you ever noticed that when you go on a diet you are always hungry? Well there is a good reason for that and it is twofold. Firstly, fat gives satiety (satisfaction) to the body and without fat in the diet the hunger signals will always flow. Secondly, the body is smart. If it does not have the essential nutrients it needs as in essential fatty acids, vitamins and minerals, then it will send out signals for you to eat more and more until you give the body those essential nutrients. Believe it or not, you have a very sophisticated body that signals you to eat when nutrient quotients are low. If you are constantly eating empty foods manipulated by man then the body will never be satisfied and neither will your hunger.

You can deduce from all of this that it is not so much the amount of fat that you are eating but the type of fat that is of most concern – once again we have the quality/quantity issue. Studies have revealed that at least 20 to 25 per cent of our daily food intake should be fats – this is not a misprint. There are tribes in Africa whose diets include up to 40 per cent saturated fat, and heart disease and cancer are not prevalent. The Zone Diet, which claims to create a state where the mind and body are working at their ultimate best, recommends 30 per cent dietary fat. Our obsession with fat is doing more harm than good to the health and wellbeing of western society.

Nature's fats are in eggs, nuts, seeds, cold pressed oils (not manipulated in any way by technology), meat, fish, butter, chicken, fruits, vegetables, grains and legumes. Nature's fats are what nature has given us; these are good fats. Man-made, manipulated fats are bad fats.

So how do you know whether a fat is natural or man-made? All margarines are man-made; all hydrogenated and partially hydrogenated oils have been manipulated by technology in some way. Most oils that sit on a supermarket shelf indefinitely have been changed in some way. These are not in their natural state, as they have been extracted from a food. The best oils to consume are the ones that have had the least processing, with the fewest additives. If you see 'cold pressed' on the label that's a good indicator that an oil has received minimal processing. You can buy olive, macadamia, almond and many other cold pressed oils. Yes, they are a little more expensive, but it's better to spend a little more on your health now than to spend thousands on health care as you get older.

Other places to find technology fats are in breakfast cereals, peanut butters, dried fruit, biscuits, crackers, confectionery, chocolate, lite and low fat dairy products. The list is endless. Not all name brands of these products contain manipulated fats – you just need to read the labels. And if you are unsure about the oil that is in a product, call the manufacturers and ask if they use hydrogenated or partially hydrogenated oils in their product. I rang a popular peanut butter manufacturer who had declared only 'oil' on the label. I asked if they used hydrogenated oil and the answer was yes. Needless to say, I don't buy their product.

Our bodies are made up of trillions of cells. Each cell has a membrane that is made up mainly of fat, with proteins embedded and sugar molecules dangling off the side for communication. The membrane helps with the passage of nutrients and other body chemicals into and out of the cell. Research has shown that if the main source of fat in the diet is hydrogenated vegetable oils, like margarine, then the membrane of the cell is not as fluid at allowing the passage of important nutrients, such as minerals, vitamins and glucose, into the cells. If the cell does not receive the right amount of nutrients it needs in order to manufacture hormones and other essential messengers and products for the body, as well as to make more cells, the body will not function at a healthy capacity and the result is disease. I find it interesting that the incidence of diabetes has increased 300 per cent in the past 20 years! We know that hydrogenated vegetable oil inhibits cell membrane function, thus inhibiting the passage of glucose into the cell, as well as inhibiting insulin receptors. The evidence is mounting against sugar being the main culprit for the diabetes epidemic. Rather, the quality of the fat we are consuming is increasingly seen as one of the main culprits. If in doubt, leave it out of your diet – it seems only prudent.

By replacing your fat intake from hydrogenated or partially hydrogenated vegetable oils, margarine, trans fats and any food that is made with these fats with good quality, nature-based fats, the quality of the cell membrane will improve. In order to avoid these fats it is very important to read food labels to check for their presence.

Here is an example of a misconception as to what are good and bad fats: coconut milk. This fabulous food is used in many dishes, but people seem to have an aversion to it because it contains saturated fat.

Recently, I was at a function with some people who weren't aware that I was a nutritionist. These people were obsessed with fat – making sure that everything they ate had a low fat or lite label. They suggested that mixing lite evaporated milk with coconut essence made a great substitute for coconut milk. I was totally blown away that people have reached the stage that they will happily eat a totally fake food rather than a natural one simply to avoid fat.

I can't stress enough that you should always choose foods from nature (even if they do contain a little more fat) rather than choose a fake manipulated food with less fat.

One final point on fats. The food industry spends a fortune developing fat substitutes. Don't be tempted to try any of these. The latest potential fat substitute is called Olestra®. This fat substitute has been approved for use in some snack foods in the USA, but not without controversy. Olestra® is synthetic fat not found in nature but manipulated and made by man. Instead of being absorbed, it goes straight through the body. The trouble is that it takes vitamins A, D, E and K along with it, as well as carotenoids. Olestra® is unlike other additives and does not come in small amounts. Instead, Olestra® will make up a large percentage of the food to which it is added. For instance, a potato chip will contain one-third Olestra®. If the loss of vitamins isn't enough to turn you away from Olestra® then this should: Olestra® taken in large quantities has the potential to cause anal leakage, faecal urgency and stomach cramps. Not a good thing to add to a diet.

Olestra® is a health time bomb. No one is certain that Olestra® is not dangerous. And it has the potential to lure people obsessed with fat into eating Olestra®-laden snack foods, with the promise that these manipulated junk foods will keep you thin and healthy. Beware!

To summarise: natural fats are in, fake fats are out. Enjoy the new experience of not having to worry about how much fat is in each food by eating a healthy balanced diet, choosing your food from natural sources and not for fat content. Then the fat you eat will be exactly the right amount.

ACTION STEPS FOR THIS WEEK

1

Start eating fat again, but only fats from nature.

2

Stay away from the fake foods manipulated to be lite, low-fat and non-fat.

3

Read all labels for the type of fat that is used.

4

Stay away from all hydrogenated and partially hydrogenated oils.

5

Enjoy the satiety, health benefits and taste of real foods and real fat.

11

GO BACK
TO BUTTER

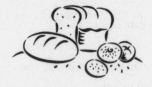

Personal growth can only begin with physical health.

After thirty years of being told that butter is bad for you and margarine is good, you're probably appalled that I could suggest that butter could be the healthier option of the two. But let's look at the facts.

Let me first tell you about the history of margarine. Margarine is the result of a process called hydrogenation. It is performed so that oils, which would normally be liquid at room temperature, are solid. In order to do this the natural configuration (cis) of the fat molecule has to be changed to a state that is never found naturally in food. This is called transconfiguration and the fats that have been changed are termed trans fatty acids or TFAs.

This hydrogenation process was patented back in 1910 and

manufacture of margarine started. By 1920 people began to substitute this new cheaper version for butter and slowly but surely there has been a swing away from lard, tallow and butter and towards margarine and vegetable oils. This is evidenced in the supermarket dairy case when you stand before the butter and margarine section. Ninety per cent is margarine and only 10 per cent butter, which brings me to the conclusion that 90 per cent of the population is eating margarine and only 10 per cent butter. This ratio was reversed only eighty years ago.

The process by which margarine is made must be seen as a money making venture on the part of the manufacturer. Therefore the oils and fats that are used are not necessarily of a high quality, otherwise margarine would be priced out of the market.

Margarine has an indefinite shelf life and to obtain this property the manufacturer subjects the fats and oils to enormous heat and to other processes including hydrogenation, deodorisation, winterisation, bleaching and refining. Products such as nickel, aluminium, hydrogen gas, benzoate dyes, colouring, artificial flavours, polyglycerol esters, vegetable gums and antioxidants are added at strategic points of the process, bringing immortality to margarine. Doesn't that sound healthy!

It is beyond my comprehension why people choose a totally artificial food as their saviour from heart disease over a natural product like butter. I believe clever advertising may be the culprit.

Let me tell you what trans fatty acids do to the body. Research has shown the TFAs suppress the immune system, cause cell membranes to leak, disrupting cell and body function, and are a major contributing factor in heart disease and cancer.

Hang on there; run that by me again! Yes, you read right. Let me briefly explain. Before margarine, we ate butter, tallow and lard. The cancer rate was 6 per cent. It is now 25 per cent and rising. Heart disease was minimal – in fact there was little death from myocardial infarction (heart attack) and now it is a major cause of death. Scientists saw this trend and found a possible culprit: man-made, manipulated fats.

Denmark and Holland have already made moves to eradicate TFAs from the supermarket shelves and thus from their diets. In fact they do not allow anything with more than 0.1 per cent TFA into the country, yet we allow margarine with TFAs in the 9 to 16 per cent range to be stocked on supermarket shelves for consumption. In the USA there is a lobby trying to eradicate all hydrogenated and partially hydrogenated fats (TFAs) from the food-processing industry. They have a long way to go. When will the English-speaking western world wake up to the dangers of technology fats?

Not all Australian margarines have high amounts of TFAs. In fact, the levels have never been as high as those manufactured in the United States, which can range from 30 to 50 per cent. But whether the margarine in Australia has lower rates of TFAs or not still does not make margarine an acceptable food to eat. It is also manipulated and contains additives and colourings.

There is also a body of evidence linking margarine to Australia's growing rate of skin cancer. The huge increase in consumption of polyunsaturated fats from margarines and cooking oils is believed to be one of the factors contributing to the increase of melanomas, although further research needs to be done to confirm this theory.

I don't wish to terrify you, just simply to point out that butter is a natural food, whereas margarine is totally artificial. Butter is better, although it does contain some additives. Just make sure you consume it in moderation, and choose an unsalted version where possible, because the salt used is usually refined. It's a simple habit to change, because butter is better in every way.

Alternatively, replace butter with a good cold pressed oil in your cooking, and use nut butters (cashew butter, almond butter, macadamia butter) on your toast and sandwiches. Macadamia butter is especially yummy in sandwiches.

ACTION STEPS FOR THIS WEEK

1

Throw away the margarine.

2

Buy butter and keep it in a covered container in the pantry for easy spreading.

3

Enjoy the taste of real food again.

12

BUY A
NUTCRACKER

*It is important to have goals, but never forget
the lessons learnt on the journey.*

This week, I want you to go nuts. Specifically, I'd like you to buy a variety of nuts in the shell, get a nutcracker and put them on the coffee table. If you're thinking 'I've got some packets of nuts – they'll do', then think again!

Nuts in their shells are much like eggs. The shell is what keeps the food inside fresh. Crack an eggshell, and the egg starts to deteriorate. Imagine if you cracked fifty eggs, put them in a plastic container without preservatives, then stuck them on the supermarket shelf for twelve months. Yuk! The same principle applies to nuts. As soon as the shells are cracked, they deteriorate rapidly. They become stale, rancid and spoiled. To avoid this, food manufacturers add preservatives to the nuts to keep them 'fresh'. The most common additives are butylated hydroxyanisole (BHA) number 320 and butylated hydroxytoluene (BHT) number 321. These are antioxidants with known adverse side effects, so why expose yourself to them?

Your taste buds can tell the difference between packaged nuts and freshly cracked nuts, so try this experiment. Taste some freshly cracked walnuts and then try the ones that come in a plastic bag – the difference is amazing.

More than just tasting better, fresh nuts (almonds, brazil, hazel, pecan, walnut, pine, macadamia and chicory) are nature's vitamin and mineral tablets. In fact, walnuts are a fabulous brain food, and I find it amusingly appropriate that they also look like a brain. They are packed with essential fatty acids, vitamins (especially E and B), phytonutrients, antioxidants, amino acids (protein), fibre and concentrated energy. Nuts provide an abundance of important minerals like calcium, zinc, selenium, phosphorus, potassium, iron and magnesium. But as each type of nut has different levels of these minerals, it's important to eat a variety of them rather than just eating one kind.

Nuts also seem to have a wonderful balance of fats. They are normally high in monounsaturated fats and have minimal polyunsaturated and saturated fats – which is nature's balance. Each time you eat a nut it is like taking a multi-goodness tablet packed with energy. And if you can buy organically grown nuts then all the better, although I find that the chemical residue of many nuts is minimal or nil and I guess that is because of the hard shell that surrounds and protects the nut. As a rule of thumb, the harder the shell the lower the chemical residue. Therefore macadamia would be on top of the list. It has also been discovered that if there are not enough minerals in the soil then the yield of the nut crop will decrease rather than the nutritional value within each nut being lower. And that's good news.

By the way, a lot of people aren't aware that peanuts aren't nuts. They are legumes. Peanuts contain 26 per cent protein, and are an excellent source of vitamin B3 and biotin. A popular way of consuming peanuts is in peanut butter. Most peanut butters these days have salt, sugar and oil added to them and more often than not it is a hydrogenated oil with the likelihood of some trans fatty acids being present. The best peanut butter is raw, freshly ground, and has been kept constantly refrigerated. However, because peanuts are grown beneath the soil, the moist conditions can cause a mould to grow on the nuts. When the nuts are not stored correctly, the mould can produce an aflatoxin, which is known to be toxic to the liver, with cases of hepatitis reported after an indulgence in peanuts. So only consume them sparingly.

There are plenty of benefits to buying nuts in their shell. For starters, they're cheaper and fresher that way. And secondly, you can't eat too many of them at one sitting if you have to crack them all first! And that's important. Try not to eat too many nuts at one time as they are a high energy source.

So this week's habit is to eat fresh nuts on a regular basis, and to buy them in their shells. Go on – get cracking!

ACTION STEPS FOR THIS WEEK

1

Buy a nutcracker.

2

Buy a variety of nuts in their shells.

3

Put them on the coffee table and enjoy the
experience.

13

EGGS – ALL THEY'RE CRACKED UP TO BE

Saturated fats and cholesterol are not the cause of
coronary heart disease. That myth is the greatest
scientific deception of this century.
DR GEORGE V. MANN

Let's get it out in the open right here and now – eggs are good for you! For thousands of years, we've been robbing nests to get them, and eggs have made a valuable contribution to the human diet. But wait a minute. Don't eggs give us high cholesterol, causing heart disease and stroke? Well that's what we've been told over the years, but I'm here to tell you that this is rubbish.

Let's first dispel the cholesterol level myth. Dr William Kannel, director of the long-term US Framingham study on heart disease, found 'no discernible association between the amount of cholesterol in the diet and the level of cholesterol in the blood, regardless of how much or how little animal fat in the diet'. That is not to say that you should go overboard with eating saturated animal fat – remember, everything in moderation – but what it does tell us is that there is no need to be paranoid about consuming these fats.

There is also some discrepancy as to whether cholesterol levels are a good indication of heart disease. At maximum only 40 per cent of people with blocked arteries and heart disease have elevated blood cholesterol levels. How do we explain the other 60 per cent that do not have elevated cholesterol levels?

So why do some people have high cholesterol while others don't? I really think it is an individual thing. Levels will rise and fall many times in a person's lifetime. When you are stressed, your adrenal glands and liver increase the level of cholesterol in your blood – and for a very good reason. Studies have shown that a low level of cholesterol impairs the body's ability to cope with physical and emotional stress. Therefore a higher level is helping the body cope with stress. This occurs because cholesterol is the building block for the stress hormone cortisol. In other words it is an old-fashioned mechanism the body needs for survival – to enable it to fight or flee.

Let us also dismiss the notion that low cholesterol levels in the blood are good. This is not necessarily so. Studies have shown that the lower the cholesterol level the more likely men are to die from suicide. There is also a possibility that the lower your cholesterol levels the higher your risk of cancer. Pritikin, the engineer and author, decreased his cholesterol levels, but got leukemia and then committed suicide. Perhaps he was missing a vital ingredient for health.

When you have your blood tested for cholesterol levels, you usually get a reading for HDL and LDL, also called respectively good cholesterol and bad cholesterol. Whoever heard of such nonsense! As if something evolved in the body for a specific reason could be bad, just because research has found it does not fit into its criteria. LDLs serve a particular purpose in the body to take cholesterol formed in the liver to the surrounding tissues for the manufacture of vital hormones. Without it we would have no sexuality, and no coping skills, or be diminished in other important products for which cholestrol is the precursor. The body is a remarkably fine working machine and when given the right foods (nature foods) and building blocks, it will run exactly as it should. We have just forgotten how innate this mechanism is.

Now that's out of the way, let's look at why eggs and cholesterol are good for you.

Apart from the cholesterol you consume, your liver and adrenal glands produce cholesterol. It helps in the manufacture of vital hormones including oestrogen (female sex hormone), cortisone (stress hormone) and testosterone (male sex hormone). Every cell in our body needs cholesterol. It's an important substance for our health. It promotes the health of the intestinal wall and is a protection against colon cancer. Cholesterol is an antioxidant. Our bodies produce a large percentage of all the cholesterol we need, and our liver regulates the levels of cholesterol in our bloodstream. But maintaining the correct balance requires a regular supply of essential vitamins and minerals, which is why we need a good diet.

On top of that, a diet high in bad fats (man-made fats) and low in fibre and fresh foods causes the level of cholesterol and other fats to change from what is normal and required for good health. Therefore you can conclude that it's not so much foods with a high cholesterol content that cause problems, but foods high in trans fatty acids found in hydrogenated and partially hydrogenated oils. In other words, man-made fats and man-manipulated fats. And we certainly eat too much of those foods in this modern society.

Eggs are like nuts – they're nature's vitamin pills. The protein in eggs is 90 per cent available to the body, compared to 65 per cent for the protein in meats. And importantly, eggs contain essential nutrients, which actually help your liver to regulate blood cholesterol levels. They also contain a unique natural substance called lecithin, which acts as a powerful fat-dissolving agent to protect the body against fat building up in the arteries. Lecithin converts cholesterol into small particles so that it can be easily utilised by your body.

Now that we've established that eggs are good for you, let's look at the downside. Most eggs today are being laid by very unhappy chooks. They lead miserable lives, are fed inferior food pellets, injected with growth-promoting antibiotics, and live under artificial lighting in tiny cages. Do you think chickens under those conditions produce healthy eggs? I think not!

Fortunately, there is an answer. There are happy chooks out there producing healthy eggs. They run around a paddock all day scratching for their food and enjoying themselves. These chooks lay free range eggs, and you'll find these delicious, nutrient-packed eggs in health food stores, selected supermarkets, and even some butchers. Better still are organic free range eggs. This means as well as the chooks being happy, they come from chemical-free farms and when supplementary feeding is required it is quality, chemical-free, certified organic grains and meals.

So, eat the best quality eggs you can find, and enjoy them raw, boiled, poached, scrambled . . . however you like. Oh, and I want to add that in 2006 the Heart Foundation finally recognised that eggs were not as bad as they first thought, and they gave the humble egg their tick of approval.

ACTION STEPS FOR THIS WEEK

1

Search out a supplier of free-range eggs or –
even better – organic free-range.

2

Start eating eggs again, raw and cooked. They
are good for you and a great source of protein!

14

EAT MORE
THAN JUST WHEAT

Be persistent, as masterpieces take time.

Do you ever suffer from any of these symptoms: bloated stomach, diarrhoea, constipation, irritability, fatigue, flatulence, burping or water retention? A lot of Australians do, but they think it's the normal state of affairs. Doesn't everyone suffer from these discomforts?

The answer is no. These symptoms often indicate that you have an allergy or sensitivity to a particular food – as increasing numbers of us do. Much of this sensitivity is due to our increasing consumption of the same foods and refined foods, which include the many products made from refined wheat flour. It also has something to do with the blood type that runs through our veins, but I'll tell you more about that later on.

The way western people eat you would think that wheat

was the only grain available. The average diet contains a large quantity of wheat in the form of bread, cereals, pasta, crackers, cakes, biscuits, pies and more. Most people would eat at least one of these foods at every meal or snack.

I want you to stop reading after this paragraph. Get a pen and paper and, using the blank table following, write down everything you ate yesterday. Then highlight all of those foods which contain wheat. Go on – do it. It will make what I am saying more clear. You will understand precisely what I am going to explain.

Your Diet

	Yesterday	Today
Breakfast		
Morning Tea		
Lunch		
Afternoon Tea		
Dinner		
Supper		

If you are having trouble, here is an example of a diet with wheat foods highlighted. (Wheat plays a prominent role in the diet of this person.)

Breakfast	• **Wheat biscuits**, milk, sugar, **toast**, butter, Vegemite, tea, milk, sugar
Morning Tea	• Tea, milk, sugar, **blueberry muffin** and butter
Lunch	• **Two pieces of bread**, butter, cheese, tomato, ham, milkshake
Afternoon Tea	• Tea, milk, sugar, **plain biscuit**
Dinner	• **Pasta**, meat sauce, parmesan cheese, salad, mayonnaise, cheese
Supper	• Tea, milk, sugar

Back again? I'm sure you found that exercise surprising. How much wheat did you find in your diet? On average, people consume wheat almost every time they have a meal or snack, and that's too much. So I want you to look for alternative grains. There are plenty of options, as you'll see in the following table.

The first column shows all the grains that are available. The top row lists the forms in which you can buy them. The further towards the right, the more processed the grain. The crosses indicate how you can buy the grain (e.g. choose rice and pasta, and you will see X which means it is available). Finding all these foods is fairly easy. Try your health food or organic food store or the health food section of your supermarket.

A simple first step is to choose a breakfast cereal that isn't made from wheat (that is if you haven't already done this). If you haven't tried the suggestions in the breakfast chapter, then try changing your cereal from wheat based to puffed rice,

Grains – Availability and Degree of Processing

Grain	Whole	Rolled	Puffed	Flour	Pasta	Bread	Crackers
Amaranth	X	X	X	X	X	X	X
Barley	X	X	X	X	X	X	X
Buckwheat	X	X		X	X	X	X
Maize				X	X	X	X
Millet	X	X	X	X	X	X	X
Oats	X	X	X	X	X	X	X
Quinoa	X	X		X	X		
Rice	X	X	X	X	X	X	X
Rye	X	X	X	X	X	X	X
Spelt	X	X	X	X	X	X	X
Wheat	X	X	X	X	X	X	X

puffed millet or corn flakes to provide some variety. Or better still, re-read the first chapter and try those breakfast suggestions. Next, choose snacks that don't contain wheat. Try fruit or freshly shelled nuts instead of cakes and doughnuts for morning or afternoon tea. If you like crackers try the ones made from other grains and top them with some nut paste.

If you're a regular sandwich eater, try using bread that isn't made solely from wheat – like rye bread, spelt bread or corn bread. And you can now buy many wheat-free and gluten-free breads from many local bakeries and stores. The same goes for the ever-popular pasta. It's now made from a variety of grains, as seen in the table on the previous page. My favourites are buckwheat (often called soba noodles) and rice pasta, and there are companies that make rice and maize lasagne sheets. Try them for yourself and you'll find one you like. And last but not least, if you eat bread with your evening meal try cutting it out.

By following these steps, you will have drastically cut down your consumption of wheat. Good luck with this one! If it takes a little longer than a week don't worry, as developing this habit entails quite a few changes to your shopping and cooking regime. But it is important, so please make the effort. Remember – a journey of a thousand miles begins with a single step. Take that first step today.

ACTION STEPS FOR THIS WEEK

1

Monitor your wheat intake.

2

Each day try substituting one wheat product
with an alternative grain.

3

If you can buy all the grains and products organically, then that would be a better option.

15

MILK – ARE YOU GETTING TOO MUCH?

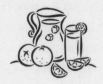

The story of survival is tied to our digestive systems.
PETER J. D'ADAMO

Before we begin this week's habit, I have a question for you. Apart from human beings, what other animal on this planet drinks milk as a food source after weaning? The answer: none. So why do we need to drink another animal's milk in order to be healthy? The answer: advertising and, for a small proportion of the world's population, the genetics to drink milk.

Do we really need cow's milk? Aren't mammals best raised on milk from the breast of their own species, then weaned? If cow's milk is so right for us why do dairy companies push the low fat version so hard, and why is moo-less milk making such inroads?

The dairy industry wants us to drink milk and consume other dairy products, so their advertising leads us to believe it's healthy and makes us feel good. But don't be fooled – drinking modern milk and consuming modern dairy foods is not the answer to good health. It is interesting to note the five highest dairy-consuming countries in the world have the highest incidence of osteoporosis.

But what about the food pyramid? Isn't dairy a main food group? Well, here's something you probably don't know: the food pyramid that is supposed to show us how much of each food group to eat wasn't designed by doctors or nutritionists or a health department, but rather by the American Meat Packers as a marketing tool to increase the sales of meat and, therefore, their profits. How scientific is that?

Why is it that we need to consume large quantities of dairy food, when our hunter-gatherer ancestors ate none? Why is it that more modern hunter-gatherers (such as Australia's indigenous peoples) consumed no dairy foods, yet were fit and healthy people with strong bones?

I know what I'm saying may come as a shock to you, but there is an easy way to prove that I'm right. For the next few weeks, try cutting down on the amount of milk you drink, the amount of cheese you eat and the amount of butter you spread on your toast, and take notice of how much better you feel. Foods have a potent effect on our bodies, and it's not until we remove a food from our diets that we realise how much it can affect us.

There may be side effects or withdrawal symptoms when you cut dairy food out of your diet. This may come about not only from the withdrawal of the food but also as a result of the withdrawal of chemical residues, antibiotics, hormone disruptors and pesticides that may be present in dairy products. If you are female, your monthly cycle could be disturbed for a short time. This is due to your hormone balance adjusting to your body's reduced consumption of saturated fats and chemicals. So be prepared.

Have you noticed how many different types of milks are available now? In the old days, there was just one kind of milk. On a recent trip to the supermarket, I counted fifteen different varieties. Sadly, none of them was biodynamic, fresh, raw milk. I believe it's the best you can buy, but unfortunately it's simply not available as it can be dangerous to those with compromised immune systems. If you are a healthy person, however, it shouldn't pose a problem. Raw milk contains the active enzymes lipase and lactase, which help in the digestion of milk. Pasteurised milk has none of these live enzymes, meaning both adults and children have a hard time digesting it. There is obviously a demand for raw whole milk as there are some innovative dairy farmers who have come up with some ways to sell theirs legally. One farmer sold his under the name 'Pets Milk' (which could only be fed to pets), while another called his 'Cleopatra's Bath Milk' (and of course you could only bathe in it). Other farmers are selling shares in their herd so that people can access raw milk.

The other process used by the dairy industry is homogenisation. This is done so the cream doesn't separate out from the milk. Now surely we haven't lost the ability to shake our milk? Unfortunately the fragmentation and pulverisation of the milk fat allows the fat to go directly into the bloodstream before being cleaned by your lymphatic system, which can cause health problems. In fact, we absorb more fat from homogenised milk than we do from butter or cream, or from milk that has not been homogenised. So for the sake of not drinking homogenised milk, just do a bit more moving and shaking.

Make sure you read the labels on your milk; some is just powdered milk with water added. Also, a note on the calcium added to milk: the best calcium for the body is the calcium that is taken up by a plant that we then eat. Many milk supplements, but not all, come from dolomite or rock sources. This calcium cannot be utilised by the body. If you don't eat rocks for your nutrition, then why would you eat rocks for your supplementation? And if the milk you're drinking with added calcium is mined from rock, then you're wasting your time drinking calcium-enriched milk.

So what's the answer? Reduce your consumption and include other sources of calcium in your diet such as sardines and salmon with soft, edible bones, oysters, and cooked bok choy, spinach, turnip greens and broccoli. If you do not wish to reduce your consumption, the best milk is that which has been tampered with the least. Ask your local health food store or organic fresh food supplier if they know where you can buy biodynamic, fresh, raw milk. If you cannot get this, then the next best is organic or biodynamic, pasteurised-only. This milk can now be found in many grocery stores.

Milk isn't the only dairy food you need to be aware of. There's butter, cheese, cream, sour cream, yoghurt and any food that contains these ingredients. Once you look, you'll be amazed how many foods contain dairy ingredients.

Butter
- If you've read the earlier chapters you will know that I suggest butter is better because it isn't manufactured in a chemical laboratory. Go for the best quality with the fewest additives. Beware of many of the soft butters – they usually use substandard oils. If you want soft butter, make it yourself. Just add a good quality cold-pressed oil to your butter in equal proportions; less if you want a harder butter and more if you want it softer.

Ghee
- Ghee is a clarified butter or pure butter fat with many of the impurities of butter taken out. It has no salt added and can be used in place of butter for many recipes.

Yoghurt
- There is a misconception that yoghurt is a fantastic health food. Yes, it once was, until it became commercialised. These days, most yoghurts have more additives than a luxury car. Go back to the traditional way yoghurt was made, then add your own goodies. Try maple yoghurt as a special treat – made from plain traditional yoghurt, with nothing added but a little pure maple syrup. Yum! Experiment for yourself.

Cheese
- Historians believe cheese was first made around 4000 years ago as a way of preserving milk. It wasn't until the 17th century that its use became widespread. Then in 1917, JL Kraft patented a method for making processed cheese. That was a sad day for our health, because now processed cheese is all you can buy in most stores. When my husband and I lived in Melbourne, we found an old Italian man who made cheese the old-fashioned way. Because it was made traditionally, it was never refrigerated, but it tasted great! Do some research in your area

and see if you can find a source of healthy traditional cheese. More and more there are boutique cheese manufacturers springing up that make cheese the old-fashioned way – seek out one in your area and start supporting them. The other types of cheese to be aware of are the soft kind – cottage, ricotta, fetta and so on. Read the labels carefully and beware of additives. Only buy the best, preferably the one which has been processed the least.

Cream
- If you can find raw cream, with nothing added, buy it. If not, the advice above applies – buy the one that has been processed the least. Sour cream is the same. That beautiful white colour is not the natural colour of sour cream so read the label and look for additives. Not that long ago there was only one cream I could buy that was pure, but once again the demand for real and pure cream is increasing and it is now more readily available.

Ice-cream
- What a delicacy! Made up of all those goodies like milk, cream, sugar and fruit. Well at least that's what it *used* to be made from. These days they mix in so many additives, I doubt they have remembered the old-fashioned recipe. I checked out one of the more popular brands and found that this is what they may add: concentrated skim milk, sugar, glucose, vegetable fat, whey powder, gelatin, natural flavour, colour 150, 160b, malt extract, food acid 330, water. Don't touch the stuff, at least not the new stuff. Go back to old-fashioned ice-cream. What is great news is that there are some small time operators out there who are making ice-cream like Grandma did and people are realising how much better it tastes.

So hunt these people out – the ice-cream makers who add nothing but natural wholefoods. The ingredients will look something like this: milk, cream, sugar and eggs. Or, better still, make your own. There are some great ice-cream makers on the market that make home made ice-cream easy. But remember this is a delicacy that should definitely be eaten in moderation. Enjoy!

The simplest way around the dairy food problem is to only eat dairy as a condiment and make sure you eat the best, what nature gave us not what technology has manipulated and changed.

Write out your food intake over the last few days and highlight anything that contains dairy ingredients. It will shock you to discover that most meals and snacks contain dairy products. Following is an example of a typical diet with the dairy components highlighted.

Typical Diet Showing Dairy Components

Breakfast	• Wheat biscuits, **milk**, sugar, toast, **butter**, Vegemite, tea, **milk**, sugar
Morning Tea	• Tea, **milk**, sugar, blueberry muffin and **butter**
Lunch	• Two pieces of bread, **butter**, **cheese**, tomato, ham, **milkshake**
Afternoon Tea	• Tea, **milk**, sugar, plain biscuit
Dinner	• Pasta, meat sauce, **parmesan cheese**, salad, **mayonnaise**, **cheese**
Supper	• Tea, **milk**, sugar

Dairy foods play a prominent role in the diet of this person.

Once you're aware of just how much dairy food you're consuming, it'll be easier to change your diet. Good luck – and don't worry if you get minor side effects. They'll pass quickly.

Now for the 'moo-less' varieties of milk: soy milk, rice milk, almond milk, quinoa milk, hazelnut milk, etc. The proliferation of these milks shows the trend in drinking less dairy. Some are healthy, while some have been heavily modified to look and taste like milk with way too many additives. There are some exceptions, but it is important to read those labels carefully or, better still, make your own. See my *Changing Habits, Changing Lives Cookbook*.

The last two habit changes have been about wheat and dairy foods. I find it remarkable that just 20 or so years ago the terms coeliac, wheat-intolerant and dairy-intolerant were not common, but it now seems that everyone knows someone who has these problems or is affected themselves. By putting some effort into using a variety of good quality foods, you will help stem this epidemic.

Following is an example that highlights both the wheat and dairy components of a diet. Most of the diet is highlighted because most of the typical western diet is heavily laden with wheat and dairy foods. If all the wheat and dairy ingredients were taken out there would be little left in the diet – perhaps some Vegemite, a few small portions of vegetables, some sugar and a bit of meat. Not enough variety for the nutritional needs of a healthy person! Using the alternatives to wheat and making dairy foods a condiment rather than a food source would leave a lot more room for fresh fruits and vegetables, good quality protein and nuts.

Typical Diet – Wheat and Dairy Components Highlighted

Breakfast	• **Wheat biscuits**, **milk**, sugar, **toast**, **butter**, Vegemite, tea, **milk**, sugar
Morning Tea	• Tea, **milk**, sugar, **blueberry muffin** and **butter**
Lunch	• **Two pieces of bread**, **butter**, **cheese**, tomato, ham, **milkshake**
Afternoon Tea	• Tea, **milk**, sugar, **plain biscuit**
Dinner	• **Pasta**, meat sauce, **parmesan cheese**, salad, **mayonnaise**, **cheese**
Supper	• Tea, **milk**, sugar

ACTION STEPS FOR THIS WEEK

1

Use all dairy ingredients as condiments rather than food sources.

2

If you choose to eat dairy foods, go back to the whole and natural form, and biodynamic where possible.

3

Be aware of the nutritional advantages of having a variety of food sources.

16

MEATING YOUR DIETARY NEEDS

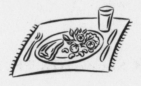

*The past does not equal your future – you have worked
all these years to arrive at this day.*

Back when humanity's most serious dietary problem was
the chance of ending up as lunch for a ferocious carnivore, our diet consisted of fruits, vegetables and grains. We
weren't ferocious enough to be great hunters, but we were
smart enough to be great scavengers. When a strong carnivore
such as a cheetah had killed its prey and eaten its fill, we would
step in and feast on the leftovers. The occasional feed of meat
was a real treat – it didn't happen at every meal.

As man progressed, we learned to kill our own beasts. But
armed with only the crudest weapons, success came only occasionally. Our diet still consisted largely of fruit, vegies and grains,
with meat an irregular supplement. As time went on we became

masters at hunting and meat became a staple in the diet but along with all the other vegetable goodies nature could provide.

It is only in the last fifty years or so that we have developed the capability and the wealth to dine on meat whenever we like. Now the average family in the developed world eats meat at least twice a day. But not only has the quantity of meat we devour changed, so has the quality of the meat. No more wild animals roaming the untamed wilderness – much of today's meat is processed, manufactured, and contains many chemicals, additives and pesticide residues.

There are 1.28 billion cattle in the world – one for every four of us. Apart from the dietary ramifications of eating meat, the production and keeping of these docile bovines is straining the planet's resources.

Cows are also inefficient converters of vegetation into meat. The production of 1 kg of beef requires the cow to eat 16 kg of grain and soy feed. In pigs the ratio is 6:1 and chicken 3:1. This equates to livestock consuming more than a third of all the world's grain.

Economically, eating meat does not work. In terms of health, eating meat has been linked to some horrendous diseases including Mad Cow disease. Nobody knows what causes this disease, whether it is a virus, bacteria or small protein. But what is suspected is animal husbandry. In the late eighties, cows, pigs and chickens were fed meat meal, which is off-cuts from butchers and abattoirs. There is suspicion that this is what may have caused Mad Cow disease. Cattle are no longer given the meat meal, but pigs and poultry continue to be fed it.

Other diseases such as heart disease, stroke and arteriosclerosis have also been linked to meat eating, especially red meat. I don't think the meat is the problem but how much we eat and of what type and quality.

Organic farming practices need to be adopted for cows, poultry and pigs. Biodynamic red meat and organic free range chickens are what they are termed. These animals are bred the old-fashioned way. The meat is free from drugs, steroids and other chemicals. I live in an area with a population of 240 000 and I only know of two places in which to buy these meat products. The demand is not high at present, but the more people become aware of choosing biodynamic meat as a healthy alternative, the more butchers will obtain and sell it. Phone your organic society to find out your closest supplier. (See appendix.)

More and more types of meats are becoming available such as kangaroo, goat, emu and crocodile. These are still basically wild meats which aren't tampered with. Let's hope they stay that way.

We are all individuals and I do not believe that genetically all of us should be vegetarians – although I do believe that some people can live a long healthy life without meat and definitely without animal products. History has shown us that our ancestors ate meat. So eating meat is not detrimental to your health. It is all in the circle of life, as long as it is not abused. What is of concern for your health is the quality and quantity of meat that is consumed.

So what role should meat play in a healthy, balanced diet and how much is too much?

A high protein diet, with a lot of flesh and dairy products, requires more calcium for body homeostasis, and if the calcium is not provided in the diet then calcium will be leached out of the bones to compensate. A high protein diet is also very taxing on the kidneys and creates an acidic environment in the body. Therefore it would be reasonable to assume that a diet with moderate protein would be a far better choice.

Protein sources are fruits, vegetables, nuts, legumes (lentils, chickpeas, red-kidney beans, etc.), seeds and grains. A complete protein is found in all flesh foods (such as red meat, white meat and fish) and eggs. As long as you consume a complete protein every day, or a variety of incomplete proteins that complement each other to form a complete protein, then you are on your way to getting enough protein in your diet. I believe that you should have variety. A typical week of eating would go something like this . . .

Monday	Organic free-range chicken
Tuesday	Organic free-range eggs
Wednesday	Rice and nuts (complementary proteins)
Thursday	Biodynamic organic beef
Friday	Fish
Saturday	Pasta and leafy vegetables, with nuts (complementary proteins)
Sunday	Biodynamic organic lamb

There is no need to be eating any more flesh than the above mentioned – you could eat less if you desire.

It is a well-known fact that fish is an important part of a healthy diet. Fish is high in protein and omega-3 oils, two important components for a healthy heart, circulatory system and brain. But there is a downside to fish and it is important that this information is not taken lightly, especially by women who are pregnant or breastfeeding.

Many fish species contain, in varying amounts, the toxic element mercury. The mercury found in fish mainly comes from ocean sediment, which is transformed by micro-organisms into methylmercury. Mercury is collected through the gills as fish breathe and through the digestive tract as they feed. This metal is then deposited within the flesh of the fish. Food processing, preparation or cooking techniques do not significantly reduce the amount of mercury within fish.

The unborn babies of pregnant women are at the greatest risk. Mercury affects the nervous system and can slow down development in the early years of life. Women should be careful about the kinds and amounts of fish they eat during pregnancy and breastfeeding.

Mercury levels differ with different fish, depending on size, location, habitat, diet and age. Fish at the top of the food chain and larger fish tend to contain more mercury than their counterparts.

Fish that contain higher levels of mercury include shark (often called flake), swordfish, barramundi, gemfish, ling, southern bluefin tuna and orange roughie. Seafood with lower levels of mercury include prawns, lobsters, oysters, salmon and tinned tuna.

For healthy adults and children, mercury from most fish is not a health risk when fish is consumed once or twice a week as part of a healthy diet. However, fish with high levels of mercury, like flake, should probably not be eaten more than once a week.

Other toxins to be aware of in fish and some types of meat are the dioxins. Dioxins are persistent organic pollutants that are formed as by-products during industrial processing, as well as being produced as a result of volcanic eruptions and forest fires. Dioxins are usually found in high concentrations in the fat of animals and fish toward the end of the food chain. Short-term exposure to dioxins can cause skin lesions and liver dysfunction. Long-term exposure to dioxins decreases the effectiveness of the immune system, can cause cancer, impairs a developing nervous system, and disrupts the endocrine and reproductive system. Fish that are caught near industrial areas or urban sprawls are more likely to have higher concentrations of this toxin than fish found in less populated areas.

This information about fish is offered merely to make you aware that there are some things that you should take into account when choosing fish, and that fish, like any food, should be eaten in moderation as part of a healthy, balanced eating regime.

Processed meats such as ham, bacon, devon and so on are just that – processed. I do not recommend any. The occasional cured piece of meat is not going to affect your health drastically but the weekly or daily consumption of these is a hazard to your health. The food additives that are used to preserve these meats are needed because without them there would be many deaths from the growth of toxic micro-organisms in the meat. But I also believe these additives should be avoided. The preservatives are: potassium nitrite (249), sodium nitrite (250), sodium nitrate (251) and potassium nitrate (252). The nitrites and nitrates may cause anaemia. This may cause difficulty in breathing, dizziness or headaches. These foods should not be given to infants or young children, as they are more susceptible to these effects. These additives also are capable of reacting in the stomach with substances called amines to form nitrosamines, which are potentially carcinogenic (cancer forming). We are all individuals, so the amount of meat eaten is also individual. If you follow the guidelines I've set out you will be on your way to better health.

And finally, when you do serve a meat or fish dish, make sure you eat it with a fresh salad. There's a good reason for this. Imagine if you left a piece of steak in the sun for a few hours – it would be putrid and stinking! Your stomach is hot (about 38 degrees Celsius) and meat takes a long time to digest. If it sits in your stomach for any length of time, it will putrefy – what a revolting thought! But fresh salad contains live enzymes, which speed up the digestive process, breaking the meat down quickly and avoiding digestive health problems. So avoid the breads and pastas and whip up a nice salad whenever you eat red meat, chicken or fish. And always eat more of the salad than there is of the meat, not by weight but by volume. And remember – all good things in moderation.

ACTION STEPS FOR THIS WEEK

1

Find out where your closest biodynamic butcher is. (See page 261.)

2

Ask your fish supplier whether they add any preservatives to the fish and where the fish are caught.

3

Have variety in all the proteins and eat them in moderation.

17

FOOD-MOOD CONNECTION

Anguish of mind has driven thousands to suicide;
anguish of body, none. This proves that the health of the
mind is of far more consequence to our happiness than
the health of the body, although both are deserving of
much more attention than either of them receive.
CHARLES COLTON

Just think about this: over the past 30 years the rate of depression and anxiety has increased enormously, particularly in the past five years. In the western world alone, depression is one of the most debilitating and expensive illnesses, costing billions of dollars a year. One in five westerners have some form of mental illness and around 6 per cent suffer serious depression. Considering most people are materially better off today and enjoy more convenience than existed just

30 years ago, you have to wonder what has caused the increase. Is it the pressures of the world, or is it a result of the foods we eat affecting the brain chemicals that balance mood, which in turn help with coping skills?

There are three main chemical neurotransmitters in the brain that help send messages from one cell to the next. They are dopamine, noradrenaline and serotonin. Dopamine and noradrenalin are the brain chemicals that keep us alert; they have a tendency to make us think more quickly and they increase motivation, mental acuity and productivity. Serotonin, on the other hand, is the calming brain chemical – it produces a relaxed, more focused, less anxious, less stressed, more euphoric feeling. Our levels of these neurotransmitters are directly related to the foods we eat.

Now I can see you reading with anticipation to find out which foods increase or decrease these chemicals, as there are always times in our life when we wish to have one or the other mood. It's quite simple really: *proteins* – such as meat, fish, eggs, freshly shelled nuts, yoghurt, cheese, legumes and complementary proteins – cause an increase in the brain chemicals for alertness (dopamine and noradrenaline), while *carbohydrates* – such as wheat, rye, millet, oats, rice, bread, pasta and starchy vegetables – cause an increase in the brain-calming chemical, serotonin.

The brain synthesises these chemicals (neurotransmitters) from the amino acids tryptophan and tyrosine. (Amino acids, which are the building blocks of protein, are also present as individual amino acids in carbohydrates.) As tyrosine is the precursor to dopamine and noradrenaline, and tryptophan creates serotonin, you would think that an indulgence of protein with these two key precursors would cause all three chemical neurotransmitters to increase in the brain, thus causing calmness with alertness at the same time. But not so – once again the ingenuity of the body is such that this doesn't happen.

The more protein you eat, the greater the tyrosine levels in your blood, thus causing an increase in the alertness chemicals in the brain (dopamine and noradrenaline). But this is not true for tryptophan. Tryptophan, tyrosine and four other amino acids enter the brain through the blood brain barrier (BBB), competitively, via the same mechanism. When we eat a protein, tyrosine and the four other amino acids become plentiful while tryptophan becomes scarce, therefore very little tryptophan can pass through the BBB. But when we eat a meal of carbohydrates, tyrosine and the other four amino acids become scarce, while tryptophan found in carbohydrates becomes the dominating amino acid, thus passing through the BBB easily with very little competition.

CHOOSE YOUR MOOD
BY CHOOSING YOUR FOOD

Calming Carbohydrates

All carbohydrates are not equal in their ability to offer mood-altering results. The best way to consume carbohydrates is in the form of whole grains and complex carbohydrates. Oats, millet, cracked wheat, buckwheat and rice are prime examples. Whole grains are broken down over a long period of time, keeping a constant flow of serotonin in our brain. To experience the maximum effect of carbohydrates on your mood, it is important to eat them without any protein.

Peppy Proteins

If you're feeling sluggish, protein power can produce the effect you want. Protein encourages the production of dopamine and noradrenaline, which produce alertness, mental energy and quicker reaction time. The effects of eating protein last about two to three hours. To maximise the 'arousal' effect of a protein meal, limit the intake of fat and carbohydrates. If you are not a good sleeper it is important not to eat protein for several hours before bedtime or you may experience difficulty falling asleep.

Neutral Fruit and Vegetables

Most fruits and vegetables are mood-neutral foods, so you can consume them without affecting your mood. If you're feeling the way you want to feel, a meal of fruit or a healthy salad might be the best option.

Sabotaging Fatty Foods

Fatty foods cause havoc with moods. An overburden of fats means digestion overload, causing a large portion of blood flow to leave the brain and be shunted to the digestive tract to help with digestion and absorption, thus causing a condition I call 'brain flag'. The brain simply stops working at peak efficiency and goes into slow mode, causing tiredness, forgetfulness, lack of concentration and all other mind-confusing, unwanted feelings. (By the way, a very large indulgent meal will also give the same symptoms.)

Antagonising Alcohol

Difficulty walking, blurred vision, slurred speech, slow reaction times, impaired memory: clearly, alcohol affects the brain and our moods. Alcoholism destroys the brain, but current research shows that moderate alcohol consumption increases blood flow to the brain, which seems to suggest a link with improved mental function. The results of the research show some specificity in the association between alcohol consumption and cognitive ability. Research at University College, London, has found that those who drink only one glass of wine a week have significantly sharper thought processes than teetotallers.

Exhilarating Caffeine

While caffeine is an addictive drug it can also be a very useful tool for changing moods and states of alertness. Scientists have developed various theories to explain caffeine's wake-promoting and mind-altering power. It seems to interfere with the chemical adenosine, which is a natural sleeping pill made by the body. Caffeine has been shown to enhance mood and increase alertness; in moderate amounts it's potent for athletes, students, brain-storming committees and the like. Used wisely, and not as an hourly pick-me-up, caffeine taken as tea or coffee can alter brain performance, making it a very useful tool.

Outstanding Omega-3 Fatty Acids

Omega-3 fatty acids found in oily fish like salmon and mackerel, as well as many nuts, like walnuts, can help stave off depression. Recent research has revealed that omega-3 is excellent for improving concentration and energy levels.

Helpful Herbs

Herbs have been used for centuries, not only for flavour in cooking but as natural remedies too. Ginger can lift the spirit, cinnamon counteracts exhaustion, camomile helps with nervous tension, while peppermint can be taken to help calm nerves and relieve anger. Basil is thought to clarify the mind, so try a large batch of pesto stirred through some healthy pasta to give your mind clarity.

Vital Vitamins and Minerals

B-vitamins play an important role in brain function. B6 helps to convert tryptophan into serotonin, vitamin B1 helps build and maintain healthy brain cells, and folic acid is also an essential brain food. Zinc is a mineral that helps keep the senses sharp as well as encouraging a healthy immune system – it is critical for proper growth and development of the nervous system.

Stimulating Sunlight

The sun inhibits a hormone in the brain called melatonin. This hormone creates a calmness in the brain and gets the body and mind ready for sleep. It is a hormone that is needed at night so it is produced when the sun goes down, but during the day exposure to sunlight will help keep melatonin at bay and enhance the alert state of the brain, as well as help get rid of the blues.

Overboard Overeating

Overeating also creates mood changes. For example, what do you want to do straight after Christmas dinner? The usual answer is have a siesta. What has happened is that your digestive system is overloaded, so some of the blood from the brain, arms and legs is shunted to the digestive system to help in the process of delivering the food's nutrients to the rest of the body. That's why when you eat too much food you either want to sleep or you find it hard to get physically motivated. If you don't digest the food within six hours or so then it begins to putrefy, releasing toxins into the blood and creating havoc with energy and mood.

You can use the principles of Food–Mood Connection in relation to sports performance. While peak performance of the physical body is important for athletes, many times the mind is the edge that makes the difference. Using the foods that cause alertness in the brain can make all the difference between winning and losing.

If you are someone who finds it hard to sleep at night, to help improve your sleep patterns it would be beneficial to have protein for lunch and carbohydrates for dinner. Stop drinking all caffeine drinks at midday, don't eat any protein after lunch and make sure you sleep in a dark room. Just see what a difference it makes when your brain is calmed down.

If you want the upper hand at a business meeting then eat smart. To keep your brain sharp and alert it is important to be aware of the Food–Mood Connection. Two basic rules are: eat very little fat and eat your protein first. So a good business lunch would be a clear soup (hold the bread and butter), then fish (without sauce) and a salad and steamed vegetables (hold the alcohol). For dessert, have fruit salad – sorry, no cake or puddings. Watch what your lunch partner eats and see who has the upper hand by the end of the meal.

Sitting down and listening to a speaker, either at a conference, university lecture or school, can sometimes become tiring. Usually, during the morning sessions most people are alert and full of questions, but after lunch the yawns start and the heads start to nod. The food that is offered at lunch is often starchy, full of breads, cheeses and other foods that cause drowsiness. My suggestion is that at morning tea, don't touch the sweet pastries; just have a cup of coffee and some fruit if they are on offer. Then at lunch choose one type of meat and salad, with coffee and fruit again for afternoon tea. Using this strategy should make a difference by keeping you alert all day, allowing the brain to take in the information needed.

If you're a shift worker, to allow yourself to work to the best of your ability it is important to manipulate the foods you eat to match when you want to sleep and when you want to be awake. Make sure that throughout your shift you eat foods to increase alertness, and then, when you are ready to sleep, eat foods that increase the brain-calming chemicals. It is also very important that when you sleep you are in a dark room. The darker the room the more abundant melatonin is, to help you sleep and heal.

With this awareness of the Food–Mood Connection, you can use your food as a powerful tool to enhance performance in all areas of life. Parents can also use these principles to help children manage their busy lives.

It intrigues me that the typical western diet is carbohydrates for breakfast and lunch, and then protein for dinner. If your moods and your sleeping patterns are not working for you, try changing and manipulating the foods you eat in order to change the brain neurotransmitters to those that best suit your needs.

From the time you wake up until approximately four hours before bed, try and consume some type of protein. For breakfast, include eggs or fish, or consume a complementary protein, which includes porridge or toast with nuts. Avoid refined breakfast cereals and starchy breakfasts like toast and jam. Snacks for morning and afternoon tea should not be muffins, cakes or cookies, but rather nuts and yoghurt, or a mix of crackers and nut butters or hummus and other protein dips. Lunch should also have some protein, like salmon, beef or chicken with vegetables. Then at night you can have pasta, rice and other high-carbohydrate meals.

ACTION STEPS FOR THIS WEEK

1

Eat protein in the morning to increase brain-enhancing chemicals.

2

Snack throughout the day on nuts, yoghurt and complementary proteins.

3

At night, eat only carbohydrates without any proteins.

18

EATING FOR YOUR
BLOOD TYPE

*Blood supplies the complex delivery and defense systems
that are necessary for our very existence. It provides a
keystone for humanity, a looking glass through which we
can trace the faint tracks of our heritage.*

PETER J. D'ADAMO

It has always been a puzzle as to why some people thrive on
dairy food, others thrive on meat, while others feel great on a
strict vegetarian diet. And why does one new, in-vogue diet work
for some people and not for others? Diet can be a bit hit and
miss unless you have the secret formula. It has always been
thought that this had something to do with race and colour due
to our ancestry. But what has become quite obvious is that
neither culture, skin colour nor place of origin automatically
guarantees selection of the perfect healthy diet for an individual.

The migration of peoples and intermingling of races and cultures throughout the ages scrubs that distinction.

We are all individuals, but we can generalise just a little and find that we can actually be grouped by our blood type. This will give you a good guideline as to the main types of foods you should be eating for your health. People who have started to take responsibility for their health by changing their diet have become attuned to which foods make them feel good, but not without some pain and effort. There is a good way to bypass the pain of trying to figure out which foods make you feel good, and that is by knowing your blood type.

Blood types have evolved just like our diet has evolved over the last million years. You see, around 50 000 years ago when we were mainly hunter-gatherers, the only blood type around was O. At this stage of the evolutionary process, meat was a fairly significant part of the diet. Then when the agricultural revolution was in full swing about 15 000 years ago, the blood type A came along. A gene mutated as a response to the changing diet (an increase in grain and legume consumption) which came about due to new agricultural practices and the domestication of animals. It was a matter of survival of the fittest. During this time people ate a lot more grains and legumes and far less meat.

Climates began to change around 10 000 years ago, and as a result there was yet another change in diet. Herders became prominent and more animals became domesticated. The diet once again began to change with an increase in meat and dairy food consumption, as well as the continuing consumption of grains and legumes. As a result of this change and the law of survival of the fittest there was yet another mutation, and blood group B emerged.

As civilisation became more sophisticated there was much movement and migration. As a result there was an intermingling of cultures, leading to the emergence of the AB blood group only 900 or 1000 years ago. To this day only a small proportion of the population has this blood group, about 5 per cent.

The change and evolution of blood types was not random but a response to food availability, climate changes, and a series of environmental events spread over many thousands of years. So it goes without saying that today your digestive system still maintains the blueprint for foods your blood type ancestors consumed.

This is the reason why protein-based diets usually work for blood group O people, vegan diets work for group A and a varied diet works for groups B and AB. It also explains why one diet is never a panacea for everyone. We are all individuals with different needs, genetically coded and chosen thousands of years ago. The old saying 'You are what you eat' takes on a whole new perspective. In actual fact it should be 'You eat what you are'.

It has been known for some time that there could be a link between diseases and blood type. For instance, a person with blood group O may have a predisposition to ulcers and inflammatory diseases such as arthritis. The possibility of these diseases could increase if you eat incorrectly for your type. The foods to enhance health are what our hunter-gatherer ancestors ate – meat, vegetables, fruit, nuts, and seeds. But this group should avoid too much wheat and grain products.

Blood type A risk factors are possibly heart disease, cancer and diabetes. The types of foods that will decrease the chances of these diseases are largely vegetarian with lots of fruit, vegetables, grains, legumes, nuts and seeds. Little or no meat should be a part of the eating regime, although chicken, turkey and seafood are OK for this blood group.

The most varied blood type is B. This group should eat a variety of foods, including meat, grains, legumes, nuts, seeds, fruits and vegetables. Dairy foods can also be tolerated better than any other blood group. The risk factors of B are that slow growing viruses can attack the nervous system if you don't eat correctly and diseases like lupus, multiple sclerosis and chronic fatigue syndrome can occur.

AB has the benefits and intolerances of both blood groups A and B. By eating correctly a strong immune system can be maintained. Most foods can be tolerated, but variety is needed.

Just to help you out here, take another look at the breakfast suggestions in the first chapter. A person who is in blood group O will enjoy and feel energetic on breakfast suggestions one and two – that is, Fruit Only and the Protein Shake – whereas a person who is an A, B or AB blood group would probably do better on the rest of the breakfasts, which have the grains. Like I said, these are guidelines but it is worth using them to avoid the pain of trial and error with foods as well as the wasted time. You probably know instinctively which foods appeal and which don't. After all, the genetic blueprint telling you which foods are right for you flows through your veins.

Evolution of Man's Eating Habits

5,000,000 years ago	**Primates** Fruit eaters
55,000 years ago	**Hunter-Gatherer** Blood type O emerged. Meat, vegetables, nuts, seeds, fruit, some grains, eggs.
25,000 years ago	**Agricultural Age** Blood type A emerged. Grains, meat, vegetables, fruit, nuts, seeds, small game meat.
10,000 years ago	**Herding and Agricultural Age** Blood type B emerged due to temperature changes. Grains, legumes, vegetables, dairy, fruit, eggs, small game meat.
1200 years ago	**Beginning of Urban Age** Blood type AB emerged. Heavy migration, mixture of all foods, some preparation.
120 years ago	**Industrial Age** Invention of hydraulic press led to more oil in the diet, refinement of grains.
60 years ago	**Chemical Age** The introduction of thousands of chemicals into the food chain.

45 years ago	**Information Age** Fast takeaway foods. Chemical additives. People more interested in what goes into their heads than into their stomachs.
10 years ago	**Low Fat Revolution** Manipulation of food to make it low fat, or sugar-free – and ten years later the nation is fatter.
Today	**Genetic Modification** Genetically modified foods and terminator technology.

ACTION STEPS FOR THIS WEEK

1

Find out your blood group.

2

Find out the blood group of your partner and family.

3

Experiment by eating those foods that are correct for your blood type and avoiding those that aren't.

19

CLEAN OUT
THE PANTRY

*Lasting change is not made without a little bit of
inconvenience, even when you replace a bad habit
with a good habit.*

Beware refined foods! They look so pure and white, but they can be horrors to your body. Many years ago, eating white flour and white sugar was a sign of affluence. These days, I'd consider the eating of refined foods as a sign of ignorance.

This week we're going to get rid of all the refined foods in your diet. Out goes white bread, white salt and white sugar. In comes good old-fashioned wholemeal flour, grey sea salt and honey. It's not hard to do – it just takes a little thought.

Most people put better fuel into their cars than they do into their bodies. Would you put low-grade or substandard oil and petrol into your car? Probably not, but most people don't think twice about putting low-grade food into their bodies. And, unlike cars, you can't go out and buy a new body if this one breaks down.

A diet high in refined foods can dictate the shape and health of your body. The lack of nutrients and the high level of additives in refined foods can put an almighty strain on your body. If it can't excrete the additives, your body deals with these toxins by surrounding them with a layer of fat or by smothering the toxin with mucus. In my opinion, cellulite is merely pockets of toxins buffered by fat particles. Once you begin to eat good whole organic foods that the body has evolved to eat and start cleaning your system out, the cellulite begins to disappear.

The second way the body combats the bad aspects of refined foods is to increase mucus production. This can increase your risk of colds, flu, nasal congestion and sinus problems. Clean up the foods you eat and you'll also clean up your sinuses.

Going from a refined food diet to a wholefood diet can be a bit of a shock to the system, especially if you try to do it overnight. This dramatic change can initially make you feel worse rather than better. But after feeling unwell for up to ten days, there's a gradual increase in strength, vitality and general wellbeing. Gradually changing the diet avoids this shock to the system.

Look at it this way – your body uses good wholesome foods just like we use soap. If we take a bath or shower every day, we're clean in a few minutes. But if we don't bathe for months, it takes a lot more time and a lot more soap to clean off the grime and impurities.

Some people recommend fasting as a good way to cleanse the body. Many people who fast find that they feel sick and nauseous for five or ten days. This is because, as the body cleanses itself, all the stored toxins in the system are released. These toxins flow into the bloodstream and then out of the body via the skin, nasal passages, lungs and urine.

The gall bladder and liver excrete excess bile (and some-times even gallstones) into our intestines for elimination. Joints that contain an excess of acid (which causes arthritic pain or gout), begin to clean themselves out. And finally, medications or chemical food additives which the body has stored in buffer zones are released and eliminated. I do not endorse prolonged fasting, but detoxifying your body with good wholesome foods is a must for good health. Think of fresh fruit and vegetables as your 'soap' – together with clean water, you can use them to wash away the toxins.

More and more frequently, direct correlations are being made between our diets and many modern-day ailments. Most people in the thirty-five to forty age group who have had diets heavy in refined foods will find themselves with one or more of these ailments: headaches, chronic infections, eating disorders, varicose veins, haemorrhoids, indigestion, stomach upsets, bad circulation, depression, exhaustion or chronic fatigue syn-drome. After years of a refined food diet, you believe that the way you feel is normal. But once you've made the switch to wholefoods, you'll have so much vigour and energy you'll won-der how you ever got by before!

There are plenty of alternatives to refined foods – some are legitimate, some are complete scams. Be careful when choosing wholemeal foods. The wholemeal pasta you like may be white pasta, which has been dyed brown. I kid you not! I remember once buying some brown bread, only to find it was white bread that had been dyed brown. It was noticeable, because they hadn't mixed in the dye properly, so parts of the loaf were still white. Needless to say, that was the last time I bought bread from that bakery! By law brown bread must contain 50 per cent wholemeal flour.

So, it's time to take a serious look at the pantry and to get rid of the nasties. Read back through the earlier chapters, and make sure that your fridge or pantry only contains good, wholesome organic foods.

ACTION STEPS FOR THIS WEEK

1

By now most of the pantry should be full of wholefoods but, if it's not, now is the time to go through your pantry and be ruthless.

2

Get rid of anything devoid of nutrition.

3

Replace all refined foods with healthy whole-food alternatives.

20

THIS GOES
WITH THAT

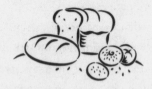

*Nothing is impossible if we believe in ourselves and
miracles. Never give up on your dreams but give praise
for everything, for all is not lost.*
BRADLEY HARRIS WOLF (AGED 14)

Over the last few years, there's been plenty of talk in the
health industry about food combining. Some deny its
potential – others believe the right combination of foods can
do wonders for your health.

What do I think? I strongly believe that food combining
promotes good health. If you doubt me, then why not try a
small experiment and judge the results yourself. But before I
tell you how to carry out that experiment, let me briefly explain
what food combining is all about.

Food combining basically means simplifying the food

groups you eat during a single meal. These days, most people eat a little of everything for each meal, jumbling together meat, dairy, starch, fats and sugars. Food combining is all about only eating one or two of these food groups during a meal, and improving your health as a result.

Now to the experiment. This will take place over your next two evening meals. On the first night, have a meal of fish, salad, carrots and beans, followed by some fresh fruit about an hour later. On the second evening, have a meal where you eat a bit of everything. Start with pâté and crackers, followed by some meat with sauce served with a baked potato with cheese and butter, a couple of slices of bread, and finish off with some pudding and cream. In other words, really put your digestive system to work.

Take note of your body's reaction to these two very different meals. How does it feel? Be aware of flatulence, burping, indigestion, bowel movements, restlessness, sleep patterns, tiredness and mental alertness. Do you feel like you need more sleep the next morning, or do you want to bounce out of bed and get going? Many people will feel a dramatic difference. For others, the difference will only be subtle. But I do believe you'll notice a difference. Once you've carried out this experiment, you need to make a decision. How do you want to feel for the rest of your life? Full of health and energy, or tired and listless? It's up to you.

The more you combine foods correctly, the more energy you'll have because your body isn't wasting effort trying to digest a jumbled mess. I have a friend who would eat cereal with milk and sugar, tea with milk and sugar, and toast with margarine and jam for breakfast every day. One day I suggested to her that she eat only fruit for breakfast to see if her energy levels would improve. She did this for about three weeks, but then decided it wasn't helping her, and went back to her old breakfast routine. That day she told me that she was so tired that she could hardly lift one foot and put it in front of the other. What had happened was that over the three week period, she was gradually getting more energy, but it wasn't noticeable to her – until she went back to her old ways and discovered how tired she used to feel from combining and eating the wrong foods.

Think back to the last time you went to a party with lots of different foods to nibble on, and you just had to sample everything. At the end of the night (and throughout the next morning) you paid for it, feeling sluggish and tired. You probably put it down to a hangover from too much drinking, but chances are you also had a food hangover. What's happening is that the jumble of various foods in your stomach is being digested very slowly, and some of it starts to putrefy and rot. Yuk! As a result, you get a bloated stomach, burping and flatulence – and some very unpleasant odours!

The benefits of combining the right foods far outweigh the slight inconvenience of figuring out what foods go together. If I go to a party with lots of yummy tidbits, I just stick to a few basic ones (usually vegetarian). This is mainly due to the fact I'm very particular about where meat comes from, as well as the food combining ramifications.

You can make food combining as simple or as complex as you want. I believe that everyone is individual, so there are no hard and fast rules. By listening to your body you will soon discover which food combinations are right for you. Watch out for those warning signs – an increase in flatulence, burping, indigestion, bloated stomach, tiredness, lethargy, irritability and insomnia. Eat the wrong foods in combination, and one or more of these warning signals will occur. There are some basic guidelines, which will help you to start combining foods correctly. The table following shows the food combinations for maximum benefit.

This simplified version of food combining is very easy to follow. Simply select a food from the vertical column, then choose a food from the horizontal column. Where the two intersect, you'll find out if that combination is good, bad or OK. For example, if you choose starches and vegetables, the combination is good. See pages 127 and 128 to find out which foods slot into the food groups.

Guide to Good Food Combinations

	Fruits	Vegetables	Starches	Primary Proteins	Secondary Proteins	Fats
Fruits	Good	OK	Good	OK	OK	Good
Vegetables	OK	Good	Good	Good	Good	OK
Starches	Good	Good	Good	Good	NO	OK
Primary Proteins	OK	Good	Good	OK	NO	OK
Secondary Proteins	OK	Good	NO	NO	NO	NO
Fats	Good	OK	OK	OK	NO	NO

Good = Enhances digestion OK = Remains the same
NO = Inhibits digestion

The body digests each of the food groups at a different speed. Eat fruit and vegies raw and by themselves, and they can be digested in forty minutes (which explains why you're hungry again within an hour if you only eat fruit). Starches last a little bit longer in your stomach, digesting in two or three hours. Proteins and fats can take up to five hours to digest. That's why when you eat fish and chips, it takes a long time to feel hungry again.

The digestion times I've just given you are for when you eat those food groups by themselves. Combine any of those food groups with another group and it either enhances the digestion process or inhibits it. Combining raw fruit and vegies with any of the food groups usually improves digestion, because fruit and vegetables contain live enzymes which enhance digestion. On the other hand, meat and fats inhibit digestion, extending the time that food stays in your stomach and allowing it to putrefy. Check the chart and see for yourself.

The main aims of food combining are to reduce the time food stays in your digestive tract, and to increase the absorption of vitamins and minerals. And the less energy your body uses to digest your food, the more energy you have to do the things you enjoy in life.

By making this change to your eating habits you'll see many benefits, so try it this week and reap the benefits. If you'd like to learn more about food combining, get hold of the book *Food Combining for Health* by Doris Grant and Jean Joice.

Foods and their Food Groups

Fruit

Apple	Cumquat	Lemon	Pineapple
Apricot	Currants	Mango	Plum
Avocado	Date	Melon	Quince
Banana	Fig	Nectarine	Raisins
Berries	Grapefruit	Orange	Tamarillo
Breadfruit	Grapes	Papaya	Tangerine
Cantaloupe	Guava	Passionfruit	Tomato
Carob	Jackfruit	Peach	Strawberries
Cherries	Kiwifruit	Pear	Watermelon

Vegetables

Asparagus	Cauliflower	Leek	Radish
Bamboo shoots	Celery	Lettuce	Red pepper
Beans	Corn	Mushrooms	Silverbeet
Beetroot	Cucumber	Onion	Spinach
Broccoli	Eggplant	Peas	Turnip
Cabbage	Green pepper	Potato	Yam
Carrot	Kale	Pumpkin	

Starches

Amaranth	Maize	Quinoa	Wheat
Barley	Millet	Rice	
Buckwheat	Oats	Rye	

Primary Protein

Baked beans	Lentils	Red kidney beans	Soya beans
Chickpeas	Nuts	Seeds	Other legumes

Secondary Protein

Chicken	Eggs	Lean red meat	Turkey
Duck	Fish		

Fats

All oils	Butter	Cheese	Lard

ACTION STEPS FOR THIS WEEK

1

Do the two evening meal experiments.

2

Decide how you want to feel.

3

Eat one concentrated food in a meal – simplify your eating.

21

SYNCHRONICITY
OF FOOD

*Until man can duplicate a single blade of grass, nature
can laugh at man's so-called scientific knowledge.*
THOMAS EDISON

While food combining on the one hand helps with digestion, there are certain food combinations that not only
help with digestion but enhance absorption and assimilation of
key nutrients.

Key micronutrients that help in the health of the body and
the prevention of disease include vitamins, minerals,
carotenoids and phytonutrients; these are found in the food we
eat. Research in this field is growing but what has been found
so far is worth noting.

Carotenoids such as lutein, lycopenes, alpha-carotene and
beta-carotene are found in many vegetables. Carotenoids have

been known to ward off many diseases, such as cancer, heart disease and macular degeneration (eye). Consuming carotenoid-rich foods – like carrots, red peppers, tomatoes, and many other red- and yellow-coloured vegetables – along with monounsaturated fat, which is found in avocados, nuts and cold-pressed nut oils, enhances the absorption and bioavailability of the carotenoids. In other words, if you have a salad, add avocado, nuts and/or cold-pressed nut oils to make sure you absorb and use more of the carotenoids in the vegetables.

What is interesting is that when you isolate any of these carotenoids they do not work as well by themselves as they do in synchronicity with other nutrients; for example, if prostate cancer cells are exposed to the carotenoid lutein alone, the single carotenoid does not prevent cancer cell growth and replication. It is the whole matrix of carotenoids and tocopherols in avocado and a salad that are necessary to kill prostate cancer cells. Researchers noted that the significant amount of monounsaturated fat in avocados plays an important role in this phenomenon.

What is amazing is that the improvement in carotenoid availability occurred even when a very small amount – as little as 40 grams – of avocado was added. Adding avocado to salad increased the average amount of absorption of alpha-carotene by 7.2 times, beta carotene by 15.5 times and lutein by 5.1 times than when an avocado-free salad was eaten. These are significant increases.

Tomatoes contain lycopenes, which are proven, powerful antioxidants implicated in the prevention of prostate, lung, bladder, cervical and skin cancer, as well as heart disease and

macular degeneration. Research shows that lycopenes in tomatoes can be absorbed more efficiently by the body if processed
into juice, sauce, paste or cooked. The chemical form of
lycopene found in tomatoes is converted by the temperature
changes involved in processing to make it more easily absorbed
by the body. If the tomato is uncooked, then adding avocado –
as in a salsa – increases lycopene and beta-carotene absorption
by 4.4 and 2.6 times respectively. Wow!

There are many nutrients that must piggyback with other
components in order for the body to absorb and assimilate
them more efficiently. Iron is one such nutrient. A number of
dietary factors influence iron absorption. The presence of vitamin C and citrate increase iron uptake. Conversely, iron
absorption is inhibited by plant phytates found in most grains
and the tannins in tea.

Iron from meat (heme-iron) is more easily absorbed then
vegetable iron (non-heme iron). But the absorption of non-
heme iron can be improved when a source of heme-iron is
consumed in the same meal. In other words, when you eat
meat, if you also eat your vegetables you'll get a double dose of
iron. While some food items can enhance iron absorption,
some can inhibit or interfere with the process. If you have an
iron deficiency problem then avoid eating the food and drink
on the right-hand side of the following table with meat, fish
and poultry. If you don't have low iron, then enjoy your meat,
fish and poultry with a variety of vegetables.

Meat, fish and poultry	Red wine, coffee and tea
Fruits: orange, cantaloupe, strawberries, grapefruit, etc.	Vegetables: spinach, chard, beet greens, rhubarb and sweet potato
Vegetables: broccoli, brussels sprouts, tomato,	Whole grains and bran
tomato juice, potato, green and red peppers	Soy products
White wine, orange juice	

For many years it has been well-known that the absorption of vitamin C is enhanced by the presence of bioflavonoids. I find it remarkable that vitamin C is found in citrus fruit while bioflavonoids are found in the citrus fruit's pith. Nature gives us synergistic combinations to help with the absorption and assimilation of many of our vitamins.

Amino acids are the building blocks of proteins. There are ten essential amino acids that we cannot make in the body but must eat in the diet. Most meat, fish and poultry have these wonderful amino acids in one package. Other foods have some, but not all of them. If there is one amino acid missing, then we call it a 'limiting' amino acid. Without that one limiting factor the whole production process comes to a stop. Combining certain foods ensures that all 10 essential amino acids are provided. The resulting combination is called complementary protein, and can be found between grains and nuts, or seeds and legumes with grains. For example, oats and walnuts, rice and lentils, wheat and almonds, and chickpeas and sesame seeds provide complementary protein.

Whenever we try to single out a vitamin or mineral and take it in supplement form, we find years later that the isolated supplement is causing more problems rather than helping our health. Food is complete; combining some foods creates even better absorption and use of nutrients than the isolation of the nutrient. Use food as your medicine for better health and well-being. Trust in the intelligence of nature and your amazing body.

ACTION STEPS FOR THIS WEEK

1

When preparing a salad, make sure it has some red, orange and yellow colours and add avocado, nuts and cold-pressed oil for increased lutein absorption.

2

Cooked or prepared tomatoes increase lycopene absorption and assimilation, so include pastes, sauces and tinned tomatoes in your cooking.

3

Add avocado to tomato to increase absorption of lycopenes.

4

Always eat food in its whole form for maximum absorption of nutrients.

5

For a complete complementary protein, combine grains with nuts, or seeds and legumes with grains.

22

THE GLYCEMIC
INDEX MADE EASY

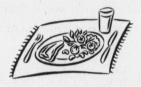

Every human being is the author of his own
health or disease.

BUDDHA

Obtaining good health is not hard and you don't need to be a rocket scientist to figure it out; you just need to use commonsense. There is no magic pill and there is no one panacea diet for everyone, as we are all unique – sometimes it takes just a bit of trial and error to figure out; what works best for your body. This week's habit change is learning about the glycemic index and using it for better health and energy.

The glycemic index is a method of measuring or ranking carbohydrates according to how they affect blood sugar levels. Until recently this rate has been ignored. The focus was more on fat levels within the blood rather than sugar, hence the low-fat diet. But you have to look at the big picture. It is important to look at all factors. It is also important to realise that the glycemic index is an average guide – not everyone will respond in exactly the same manner, and when foods are combined the glycemic rate will vary significantly.

The lower the glycemic index, the more advantageous the food is to balancing blood sugar levels and, as a side effect, blood lipid levels. With high glycemic index foods, the chances are increased of spikes in blood sugar levels from extreme highs (hyperglycemia) to extreme lows (hypoglycemia), and that's where we come unstuck. The art of keeping blood sugar levels constant, with the help of the two hormones insulin and glucagon, is part of preventing diabetes and heart disease.

The glycemic index basically measures rate of digestion (how long it takes for food to break down in the stomach, thus allowing sugar to enter the bloodstream). Foods containing carbohydrates that break down quickly during digestion have the highest GI as they send sugar into the blood quickly, causing a dramatic increase in blood sugar levels. Conversely, foods that contain carbohydrates that break down slowly have a low GI, as they release glucose slowly into the bloodstream. Both types of food have advantages – but it's best to minimise high glycemic foods.

From this, it's not hard to figure out which foods are conducive to stable blood sugar levels and which are not. Most breakfast cereals, sweets, soft drinks, white bread and most highly refined carbohydrate foods have a high glycemic index, while many fruits, vegetables, some grains, nuts and lentils have a low to moderate GI. However, there are some surprises.

Over thousands of years our diet has changed, but slowly. It is only since the introduction of high-speed, steel roller mills for grinding grains (during the Industrial Age, around 100 years ago) that the glycemic index of many foods began to increase, due to processing. And in the last 50 years, the dramatic increase in the number of high-fat takeaway and fast foods available, coupled with the low-fat revolution of foods with higher sugar content, has increased the amount of high glycemic food consumed.

This continuous eating of high glycemic carbohydrates places enormous pressure on the body's ability to keep producing large amounts of insulin in order to control blood sugar levels. The body must produce large amounts of insulin, which creates insulin resistance followed by insulin exhaustion, which leads to diabetes, hypoglycemia, obesity and heart disease.

There is much evidence that what we eat affects behaviour, mental capacity, performance and overall health. With the incidence of diabetes increasing at an unprecedented rate, it is vital to be aware of the glycemic index in order to try to prevent this lifestyle disease. In brief, a diet of lots of fruits and vegetables, fresh meat, both red and white, nuts, whole grains, healthy fats and some occasional treats will go a long way in providing a positive and healthy outcome.

The glycemic index of foods is a guide to help with everyday healthy choices, but it really just reinforces that the processing and chemical and physical manipulation of many foods has been a disaster for health. By going back to an old-fashioned diet, where fresh fruit, vegetables, meats, whole grains and some quality dairy form a large part, then we are not only following the glycemic index diet, but also the good points of healthy eating.

ACTION STEPS FOR THIS WEEK

1

Start eating more wholefoods, without refinement.

2

Become aware of the glycemic index of the foods you eat.

3

Make sure the majority of your carbohydrates are low-GI, by eating non-processed foods.

23

BALANCING PROTEINS AND CARBOHYDRATES

A man's health can be judged by which he takes two
at a time – pills or stairs.
JOAN WELSH

Having a balance between protein and carbohydrates is more sensible than eating an extreme diet of either. The proponents of the high-protein diet and the high carbohydrate, low-fat diets have been at loggerheads, each claiming theirs is the best diet for weight loss and health. I'm often asked what I think of the high-protein diet, and my reply is this: I know that protein and fat are important, and I also know that a diet devoid of fruit, vegetables and grains cannot be supplying all our nutrient needs.

What is interesting is that the high-protein diet was first designed to reduce the incidence of seizures in children with epilepsy. But because the diet was hard to maintain, and some children showed signs of cardiac irregularities, it was discontinued as a mainstream treatment.

A high-protein diet changes the body's metabolism. Metabolism is the process by which cells convert nutrients into energy after food is digested and absorbed into the blood – the higher your metabolic rate, the more quickly food is converted •into energy.

The decrease in carbohydrates of the high-protein diet causes glycogen stores (carbohydrate food stored for energy) to become depleted within 24–48 hours. This causes fat to be released into the bloodstream. This fat is then taken to the liver where it is converted into ketones. The body, including the brain and muscles, is forced to use ketones instead of glycogen for energy. Consequently, it goes into a metabolic state called 'ketosis', causing a decrease in metabolic rate. This is the body's wisdom taking over to save fuel in this time of starvation and a sure indication that your body is not getting what it needs. In fact, three weeks into ketosis the metabolic rate will have decreased by 9 per cent, and after six months it will be down by 24 per cent. A decrease in metabolism is not what we are trying to create on a lifetime diet.

When the body is in ketosis, the blood becomes more acidic, so disposing of the excess ketones increases the need for water, leading to dehydration if sufficient water intake is not maintained. Ketosis leaches potassium, calcium and sodium from the bloodstream. These three important elements are the main players in the correct working of the heart; in particular, potassium has a vital role.

In a recent study where the participants were on a high-protein low-carbohydrate diet, it was found that 20 per cent had heart problems, including heart attacks, strokes and arrhythmias. In one study in the US, 60 people died while on a low-carbohydrate, liquid protein diet – which brings to mind protein powders.

With the increased popularity of protein as a main food source in the diet, protein powders are being consumed without regard for their components. Most protein powders are, in essence, made of soy protein isolate, and vitamins and minerals created in a chemical laboratory and not by nature, thus adding their own health problems, including excessive aluminium, increased xeno-oestrogens and non-bioavailability of nutrients. The unwitting consumers are part of an unsupervised experiment where the results may not be known for many years. Are you willing to take the risk?

Let's take a look at the Atkins Diet, the most famous of the high-protein diets. During the two week 'induction' phase, when calories are reduced, there is not much change in the percentage of protein consumed compared to a normal western diet, but carbohydrates are almost nil and intake of fat increases to a whopping 65 per cent. You could almost call it a high-fat diet rather then a high-protein one. The diet is extremely high in fat, vitamins A and B12, phosphorus, sodium and potassium, and very low in fibre, vitamin E, iron, magnesium, calcium, thiamine and carbohydrates.

During the ongoing or 'maintenance' phase of the Atkins Diet, fat remains high, protein remains at about 30 per cent, and very few carbohydrates are introduced. Studies have shown that a diet lacking in fruit and vegetables increases the risk of cancer of the colon, breast, pancreas, lung, stomach, oesophagus and bladder. Low fibre consumption is never a healthy choice.

Without sufficient fruit, vegetables and especially grains in the diet, it is almost impossible to obtain an adequate amount of the essential trace mineral selenium. We know that selenium, a mineral essential for cancer prevention, is already deficient in many western diets, but without organic whole grains in the diet, selenium levels drop dangerously low, affecting the thyroid, ovaries, prostate, heart and brain.

Thirty years ago, while everyone was focusing on a low-fat, high-carbohydrate diet, people forgot about protein. The whole premise of the low-fat diet was to eat a diet low in animal fats, especially – not to replace the fat with sugar. Nor was the intention to eat large portions of low-fat products. The message was to reduce fat intake and eat more fruit, vegetables and whole grains as part of a healthy diet. The low-fat diet was misunderstood. We went overboard and the result was an increased incidence of heart disease, escalating cancer rates, a 300-fold increase in the incidence of diabetes, and a society that now has more than 50 per cent of the population obese or overweight – in all, a very unhealthy group. Are you willing to make a similar mistake by going to the other extreme?

From the above information, it seems that by being extreme in a diet you may decrease weight in the short-term, but you will not create a healthier body. Western society seems to take one aspect of research and twist it till it suits popular demand. Then, as time passes, the real ramifications of such foolhardy actions become evident.

Let's go back to something in between: a diet that has moderate amounts of protein, fat and carbohydrates. A diet that our hunter-gatherer ancestors ate – meat, vegetables, fruit, nuts, seeds, eggs and grains. Why make it so complicated? Are we so obsessed with the desire to be thin that we have lost sight of the need to be healthy?

It's time to stop all the nonsense and get back to normal eating. I believe people intuitively know what is right, but they are just too busy looking for a quick fix. The only fix that works is a change in lifestyle for a lifetime.

ACTIONS STEPS FOR THIS WEEK

1

Accept that there is no quick fix.

2

Avoid extreme quantities of any food or food group.

3

Enjoy a balanced diet with moderate amounts of fat, protein and carbohydrates.

24

THE SOYBEAN –
HEALTH OR HAZARD?

What gets us into trouble is not what we don't know.
It's what we know for sure that just ain't so.
MARK TWAIN

In this day and age it's easy to become a vegetarian – people are more knowledgeable, and the soy industry has created numerous products to enable vegetarians to obtain their daily protein. From the humble soybean we have soy flour, tempeh, tofu, soy milk, soy sauce, miso, soy cheese, soy burgers, soy mayonnaise, and even soy ice-cream.

At first this seems like a good thing, but for the last five years there has been a groundswell of negative publicity about soy, as well as a proliferation of research and new discoveries that are worth looking at. It seems soy, like many other foods I talk about, has become a victim of science and technology trying to 'improve the food' to get the most out of it financially, creating problems. While I believe soy is inherently a good food when cooked correctly and eaten in moderation, it is what we have done to the humble soybean that has created the problems we are now seeing.

Soy was traditionally used in Asian countries, but never in generous amounts. It was often used by the less affluent in times of scarcity and then only eaten after undertaking a painstaking process (lengthy fermentation) to destroy the toxins and anti-nutrients. Asians consume soy products in the form of tofu, miso, tempeh, fermented soybeans, boiled soybeans and soy milk (a very woody, bland product, not the sweetened, flavoured and chemicalised concoction sold in western grocery stores). The estimated amount of soy protein consumed from these sources is about 7 grams per day. Asians generally only use small portions of soy to complement their meal. It should also be noted that soy is not the main source of dietary protein for Asians.

On the other hand, many vegetarians in western society think nothing of consuming 220 grams of tofu and a couple of glasses of soy milk per day, two or three times a week, well in excess of what Asians typically consume.

Soy, which was once a minor crop, was not termed a food but rather an industrial product. It has now become a major food crop, and the last 20 years have seen a proliferation of soy products and by-products that dominate the market. More than half of packaged foods on grocery shelves now contain soy, in the guise of soy flour, textured vegetable protein, partially hydrogenated soybean oil, soy protein isolate and vegetable oil. Check the labels. Cake mixes, chips, crackers, cookies, margarine, infant formulas, meat substitutes and bread all contain soy in some form. Unbe-known to most of us, soy now plays a major role in our diet.

The chief concern is that mostly we are not choosing to eat this amount of soy; it is being imposed upon us. We face the risk of mega-dosing on soy, possibly causing more food sensitivities and health problems – the same scenario we have already seen with wheat and dairy. This is not about scaremongering, but rather making you aware that this food, which was not in our diet 20 years ago, is now there in increasing amounts.

Not only is soy in our diet in greater amounts, there are cer-tain dark sides to the soybean that need to be addressed. Soy contains potent enzyme inhibitors that block the action of trypsin and other protein-digesting enzymes. They can pro-duce serious gastric distress, with reduced protein digestion causing chronic deficiencies in amino acid uptake. Soybeans also contain haemagglutinin, a clot-promoting substance that causes red blood cells to clump together. Together, trypsin and haemagglutinin cause growth retardation.

Soybeans are also high in phytic acid, present in the bran or hulls of all grains. Phytic acid can block the uptake of essential minerals, such as calcium, magnesium, copper, iron and espe-cially zinc, not only found in the soy but also other foods you consume with soy. The phytates in soybeans are highly resist-ant to normal phytate-reducing techniques such as long, slow cooking. Zinc malabsorption is a major concern as it is needed for brain and nerve function.

Other parts of the soybean that are of particular concern are the endocrine-disrupting isoflavones, also known collectively as zeno or phyto-oestrogens. In 1991, a team of Japanese scientists found that two tablespoons of soy per day for one month resulted in a significant increase in thyroid-stimulating hormone. Goitre and hypothyroidism appeared in some of the subjects and many complained of constipation, fatigue and lethargy. Some studies have gone as far as saying that soy may increase the chances of oestrogen-dependent breast cancer. You have to wonder what these phyto-oestrogens are doing to children and men.

The most serious problem with soy may be its use in infant formulas. 'The amount of phyto-oestrogen that is in a day's worth of soy infant formula equals the amount of oestrogen in five birth-control pills,' says Dr Mary G. Enig, president of the Maryland Nutritionists Association. She and other nutrition experts believe that exposure to high amounts of phyto-oestrogen in infancy is associated with early puberty in girls and retarded physical maturation in boys.

While soy producers try to get rid of its anti-nutrients, in the process they destroy many of the nutrients. Miso, tofu, tempeh and other fermented soy products are by far the superior soy foods.

For me the most frightening of soy products is soy protein isolate. This is something you cannot make in your own kitchen. It is made in an industrial factory, using alkaline and acid washes with very high temperatures, high pressure and spray drying for the final product. Nitrites, which are potent carcinogens, are formed during the spray drying, and another toxin is formed during the alkaline processing. Numerous artificial flavourings, particularly MSG, are added to soy protein isolate and TVP (Textured Vegetable Protein) products to mask their natural taste. In some studies, the consumption of soy protein isolate increased requirements for vitamins E, D, K and B12 and created deficiencies in calcium, magnesium, manganese, molybdenum, copper, iron and zinc. Soy protein isolate is the key ingredient in many baby formulas, protein powders, protein bars and soy foods that imitate meat and dairy products. Please check your products and avoid this insidious ingredient.

We naively believe that the foods on our shelves are safe, but they may only be 'edible'. While I believe a small amount of soy occasionally can be good for our health, we need to be very aware of how much we are eating, especially in light of current research and knowledge. I strongly urge anyone eating soy products or drinking soy milk – that means just about everybody who buys food in a supermarket – to find out what they can about soy and its by-products.

ACTION STEPS FOR THIS WEEK

1

Read all ingredient labels in your pantry.

2

Find products in your grocery store that are free from soy products.

3

Reduce your consumption of soy.

25

JUICED
ENOUGH

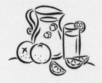

*If you don't take a little bit more time and money now
for your health, you will have to take a lot more time
and money later for illness.*

Next time you're in the supermarket, take a look at the
fruit juice section. Fifteen years ago, you would have
found orange juice, pineapple juice and perhaps tomato juice.
But today there are literally hundreds of different kinds of
juices to choose from, ranging from tropical guava cocktail to
summer berry surprise. That level of growth tells you that Australians are drinking a lot more fruit juice. And that's got to be
good for us, hasn't it?

The answer is no. The natural way to enjoy fruit is whole
and fresh, when it contains lots of healthy fibre and natural
ingredients. With most fruit juices these days, all you're getting

is a solution of colours, additives and flavourings with very little real fruit – at least that seems to be the case for the majority of them. This lack of fibre and high sugar content causes a rapid rise in your blood sugar levels followed by a sudden fall – definitely not the way to get sustained energy throughout the day. In brief, it's better to eat a piece of fruit and drink a glass of water, or squeeze your own juice.

If you must have fruit juice, at least choose the best one possible. The key to doing that is to read the label. Let's take a look at the label for a popular fruit juice drink. Under ingredients the label tells us that this particular fruit juice contains the following: reconstituted juice; puree; sugars; food acid 330; vegetable gums 466, 440; flavour; colours 102, 122. Contains 25 per cent fruit juice. No preservative added, no artificial flavouring. What does it all mean?

Let's start with the numbers. Food acid 330 is citric acid, which prevents the discolouration of fruit. In excessive amounts it can cause erosion of the teeth, so beware with young children. Vegetable gum 466 is caramelise sodium CMC, a thickening agent which is usually safe, but may cause intestinal obstruction. And 440 is pectin, a gelling agent which can cause flatulence (wind) or intestinal distension. Colours 102 and 122 are food colourings – yellow and red respectively. They are azo dyes. Asthmatics or people who are sensitive to aspirin often have negative reactions to these azo dyes, including skin rashes and purple patches, hay fever, breathing problems and blurred vision. It has recently been suggested that these dyes may be responsible for hyperactivity and wakefulness in small children at night, so if your kids aren't sleeping, these dyes may be the reason why.

But wait – there's more! You'd think that when the label says 'no added preservative' that would mean the juice contains no preservatives. But you'd be wrong. When they say 'no added preservative' it means preservative has been added, but only to a certain legal limit. And what about 'no artificial flavouring'? Well, that tells us that a flavouring has been added – a natural one. So how does the food industry define 'natural'? Food Standards Australia New Zealand has no guidelines for the term natural in most foods. There have been drafts made up, but no policies created. Therefore the food may be derived from a natural source, but after many processes it may not be in its natural state.

The same applies to sugar content. The words 'no added sugar' do not mean that there is no sugar in the product. They mean that sugar has been added up to the legal limit (around 4 per cent of the juice's content).

Sorry to burst your juice bubble like that, but you need to know that the only fruit juices which contain no additives are the ones you squeeze yourself or the ones that are squeezed at the grocery store in the fruit and vegetable section. Personally, I prefer a glass of water, with plenty of ice cubes and a slice of lemon for flavour – it's very refreshing. If you must drink a commercially prepared juice, choose the one with the lowest number of additives, and always dilute it 50 per cent juice to 50 per cent water if not more. If I ever give my children juice I use it like cordial – 20 per cent juice to 80 per cent water.

I explained this whole juice scenario to a friend once. A couple of days later she rang me to say that she had found the perfect juice. I asked her to bring me the container. I looked at it and it seemed pretty good. There was some vitamin C added, as this is law in fruit juices. But I was puzzled why it had a shelf life of twenty-one days. I presumed there must have been a preservative in the packaging. Totally bewildered I rang the manufacturer for the answer. It was revealed to me that the juice had been heated at a very high temperature (ultra pasteurisation) for a short period of time. The only vitamin that is recommended by the food standard authority to be tested after this process is vitamin C. There is still some vitamin C available, but what about the other nutrients and phytonutrients that are heat sensitive and lost in the process to some extent? I don't believe these juices are the answer. So play it safe – squeeze your own fruit juice and drink it immediately for maximum nutrition.

There are many juice bars springing up around the place, including franchises and one-offs. You can find them in shopping centres, travel stations and airports. It is important when you ask for your juice that you realise some of the juices will be commercial. If you ask for a fresh apple, beetroot, carrot and orange juice, the apple and orange portions may be commercial whereas the beetroot and carrot may be freshly squeezed. Ask at the time which of the juices will be fresh. Juice bars also serve smoothies. I ordered one not long ago at a juice bar because it said it had blueberries, strawberries, raspberries, fresh apple juice and gelato, in that order. I watched the attendant put the ingredients into the vitamiser: three large scoops of gelato, commercial apple juice, one strawberry, three raspberries and two blueberries. I was horrified. If I hadn't watched – as probably many people don't – I wouldn't have known. (It didn't taste nice and my daughter ended up throwing it away.)

Once again, where commercialisation takes over, it seems to destroy the essence of what the food is all about. Beware and make sure you are getting the real deal.

ACTION STEPS FOR THIS WEEK

1

Start diluting the juices – ultimately to 80 per cent water, 20 per cent juice.

2

Eventually cut processed juices out of your diet.

3

Choose water to quench your thirst.

26

THE ORIGINAL
IS STILL THE BEST

*People who succeed from the depths of despair make their
physical body better first.*

Diets. There are so many of them out there, it's incredibly
confusing. Protein diets, low-fat diets, starvation diets,
fruit diets. They all claim to be wonderful, yet they all conflict
with each other. It's a maze of ideas, fads, half-truths and hype.
But every now and then you'll stumble across an idea so simple
that it makes sense among the thousands of diet suggestions.
This week's habit is one of those ideas. It's a great rule of thumb.

Eat food as close to its original source as possible, and if you
don't know its origin, don't eat it. Let's take an example: the
popular snack food, Twisties. Did you know that the main
ingredient in them is corn? Unfortunately, it's not the only
ingredient. There are plenty of additives. You could get one

step closer to the original source by eating plain corn chips. Better still would be corn bread. Even better than that, corn on the cob. Another example where you can exercise choice to get closer to the original source is Burger Rings. They're made from rice – plus a cocktail of additives. A better choice would be rice crackers. Better still, rice.

Here's a quick quiz for you. Name the original source of these popular foods: black salted spreads; margarine; fruit roll-ups; protein powder; devon. If you can work out what they were originally made of, I'll eat my hat (and it would probably be more nutritious!).

Are you getting my drift? The more processing a food has gone through, usually the less nutritious it is. The closer the food is to its original form, the better it is for us. When foods are processed into an artificial state, our bodies can't use them as effectively. Sometimes it can even make that food more dangerous. For example, bran is one part of the wheat grain. We isolate the bran from the other parts of the grain and eat it. Without the other components of the wheat grain, bran can cause bowel irritability and spasms. Yet as a whole grain, wheat works as a soothing fibre promoting rhythmic peristalsis (normal movement) of the bowel.

But what about these new 'wonder foods' which keep coming onto the market: foods with a single calorie, or foods that stop fat being absorbed into the body? They don't seem to originate from any kind of food! These 'foods' are definite no-no's. Their magical properties appeal to a world looking for quick fixes. But I'm afraid there are no short cuts. The pursuit of health is an ongoing, lifelong process. You either spend a bit of time now looking after your health or you spend a lot of time later in life looking after your illness. In other words you either eat to live and be healthy or live to eat and be sick.

So this week, your task is to think before you eat. Before you put a piece of any food into your mouth, ask yourself what its original source is. Could you be eating something closer to the original? Remember that the original is still the best.

ACTION STEP FOR THIS WEEK

1

Think before you eat, and ask yourself two questions:

Do you know the original source of the food you are about to put into your mouth?

Can you move closer to the original source?

27

FORGET

ABOUT CALORIES

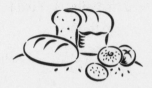

The power to change is within.
BRADLEY HARRIS WOLF (AGED 14)

This week's habit change is one you'll love. If you have one of those calorie counter books, I want you to pick it up, walk to the nearest rubbish bin, and throw it in.

There! If you've desperately tried to lose weight by counting calories, that was probably the most satisfying thing you've done all day. Now let me tell you why I suggested it.

Counting calories is a complete waste of time. Why is it that some people can consume copious amounts of calories and still maintain their weight and health, whereas the next person only has to look at a chocolate cake to put on a kilo? According to the National Health & Medical Research Council's recommended daily intake for energy, a thirty-year-old woman can consume an average of 2020 calories (8500 kilojoules) a day and maintain her present weight level. If she consumes this energy through nutrient-rich foods such as fruit, vegetables, meat or fish, grains and nuts, she is sure to get enough nutrients to run her body effectively. However, if she chooses to eat refined, processed foods she will consume enough energy, but insufficient nutrients to keep her going. What science has failed to tell us about these calculations is that there is more to the human body than just getting energy (calories/kilojoules) out of food. The truth is that despite what everyone tells us, calories are not the true value of food once put into the human body.

If you don't already know, here is a short history lesson on how these measurements of food value came about. Calories are measured by a simple machine called a bomb calorimeter. Food is placed inside, exposed to a high pressure of oxygen, and then ignited. As the food burns, the heat released can be measured in calories. As well as this process, the food is measured by what are called Atwater Factors – a process invented in the late 1800s to allow for human body mechanics.

These food values are now archaic, and are being misused. They were originally designed as a guideline for groups of people, not as the only food-value measurement for an individual. People are all different – both outside and inside. Your body will not necessarily react to a nutrient, a food or a toxin in the same way as someone else's will.

Calories are not the only value of a food. I am appalled when I see potatoes, corn, peas, avocados and bananas taken off a diet because of their high calorie content. What about the other aspects of these close-to-nature foods? What about the fact that they can enhance digestion, reduce absorption of fats, and enhance vitamin and mineral absorption? These foods have advantages that cannot be found in a diet soda drink with only one calorie.

So, if counting calories isn't the way to reduce weight, what is? The key is to change the metabolic rate of your body. Our metabolic rate is governed by a part of the brain called the hypothalamus, which also regulates body temperature. The ability of the hypothalamus to change the metabolic rate varies with each individual. Basically, it works like this: if you consistently eat a moderate amount of food, and regularly do a moderate amount of exercise, the hypothalamus sets a moderate metabolic rate for you, so that you maintain a sensible body weight.

But let's look at someone who is constantly dieting or skipping meals in an attempt to lose weight. First of all, you need to understand that our bodies have a strong survival instinct. If you eat less, the body goes into survival mode by decreasing the amount of calories it burns, by slowing down the metabolic rate. That was great a thousand years ago when food was scarce each winter, but for someone trying to achieve a model figure today, it's a nightmare.

Because of this survival mode, constant dieting will make you fat. The more you diet, the lower your metabolic rate becomes, and the fewer calories you must consume to lose weight. But if you can reset your metabolic rate to a faster pace, you can maintain or lose weight. Because we are all individuals, there will be variation, but the three major factors affecting metabolic rate are time, exercise and eating.

Time

I know – in this day and age, time is a commodity we are all short of. But as I've said before, you can spend that time now to be healthy, or you can spend it in later years being sick.

The body needs time to adjust the metabolic 'thermostat'. A conservative estimate is between six months and a year, depending on the gusto with which you tackle this change. The body can lose weight while this adjustment is being made, but it will happen slowly. I know a year sounds like a long time, but how long have you put up with feeling unhappy, unhealthy and overweight? Two years? Five years? Ten years? If you can put up with that, you can be patient for six to twelve months to feel great for a long time. Many of our weight and diet problems are related to our wimping out and choosing the quick fix – the instant frozen meal, the fast food takeaway and the fad diet. Quick fixes do not work. In fact they make the problem worse. Changing your metabolic rate isn't an instant solution, but be patient and give your body time, because *it will work!*

Exercise

This is another key ingredient in changing your metabolic rate. Some people love exercise, and some detest it. If you fall into the latter category, please bear with me.

Since the beginning of time we have exercised. As hunter-gatherers we were either being chased by a sabre-toothed tiger or running after a mammoth for our dinner. When the agricultural revolution kicked in there was constant physical activity out in the fields. The herding population walked vast distances with their herds and occasionally made a sprint for a runaway stray. When the industrial revolution came into full swing there was a lot of heavy lifting and manual labour. It is only since the sixties that we spend more time sitting in front of the computer, television or video screen, and we have gadgets to do everything. As a result we need to go out and do some sort of physical activity. You see it is in our genetic blueprint that exercise must be a part of a healthy lifestyle.

Researchers at Stanford University experimented on a group of volunteers by putting them on a moderate, steady exercise program. They began with brisk walking, then over a period of time they worked up to four to five jogs each week. The fact that exercise burns calories is no surprise. But what might surprise you is that, as time went on, the joggers began eating more and more food without increasing their level of exercise. In other words, they were consuming many more calories than their exercise was burning off. But even though they were eating more, they didn't gain weight. After six months, they were eating 300 to 400 more calories (1260 to 1680 kilojoules) each day over and above their activity level, yet they had lost 7 per cent of their body fat. And after two years they were still eating more, but maintained their weight. Why? Because the exercise had reset their metabolic rate to a higher level, allowing them to consume more without putting on weight. That's good news!

It doesn't matter what kind of exercise you choose, as long as it fits your lifestyle and you enjoy it enough to continue over time. Swim, walk, run, ride a bike, do aerobics. Variety will stop the boredom and let you enjoy it. To change your metabolic rate, you should exercise four to five times a week; do it with a fair amount of energy and gusto; and spend a minimum of thirty minutes each day on your exercise session.

Current trends are going away from the personal trainer and more to groups exercising together. I walk with several girls; we commit to each other that we will meet every morning at 5.00 a.m. The commitment makes you get going and we have some great laughs as we exercise.

Eating

The final ingredient is the most important in resetting the metabolic rate – eating. At no time should your body think that it needs to go into survival mode. Even if you're on the run, don't miss a meal. Grab an apple or a banana so that your body doesn't slow down its metabolic rate. The type of food you eat is very important, as you've already discovered throughout this book. Isn't it great to hear you have to keep eating? I bet this is a first in the diet industry!

So if you want to lose weight without gaining it back again, throw your calorie counter away, start exercising and eating moderately, and change that metabolic rate. You'll find your health and your weight will look after themselves.

ACTION STEPS FOR THIS WEEK

1

Throw the calorie counter away.

2

Start to reset your metabolic rate.

3

Time + Exercise + Eating = Increased
Metabolic Rate

28

THE
MAGIC FORMULA

*If we long for kindness we need to be kind, if we yearn for
truth we must be true to ourselves, for what we give of
ourselves is always reflected back.*

It's great to know what foods to eat, but the next question is how much of them to eat. You can spend ages weighing food, counting calories and calculating fat, but who has the time and interest to do that? So to bypass that entire hassle, I've developed a great habit called the 2–2–4–4 habit. If you're following the habits you've read so far, you may find that you're already using this technique, but it's a great way to check that you're on the right track.

Here's how the 2–2–4–4 habit works. Every day, you eat two protein, two starch, four fruit and four vegetables. This rule applies whether you weigh 55 kilos or 105 kilos. The numbers represent portions. So, if you're a big man who eats a lot, you might consume two buckets of protein, two buckets of starch, four buckets of fruit and four buckets of vegetables. A smaller eater might consume two fistfuls of protein, two fistfuls of starch, four fistfuls of fruit and four of vegetables. I realise this analogy is extreme, but I'm sure you get the picture. This is a much easier way to measure and control your intake than counting calories or weighing foods.

The general idea is to have variety within all these food groups. Proteins include red meat, fish, poultry, nuts, seeds, eggs, yoghurt, legumes, some cheeses and complementary proteins (e.g. grains and nuts, legumes and grains, grains and seeds, or lentils and nuts). I recommend that each day you have protein from an animal source (if you're not vegetarian or vegan) and protein from a plant source. If you're a vegetarian, then you must vary the protein combinations and legumes you consume. See the food combining chart in chapter 20 (This Goes With That).

Starches are all the grains – oats, wheat, rice, millet, rye, triticale, barley, maize, quinoa, spelt, amaranth and buckwheat. As well as the original grain, they're found in cereals, pasta, breads, biscuits, muffins, cakes, crackers and flours. Starch is the one food that's eaten in great excess when compared with the other food groups, as it seems every meal contains some form of starch. Look back at the chapter on wheat, or write down what you ate yesterday, and you'll see this is true. For a lot of people, breakfast is cereal, lunch is sandwiches, snacks are biscuits, crackers or muffins, and dinner usually includes bread, pasta or rice.

So starches are the food group to watch – two portions a

day is plenty. Breakfast and dinner are the best times to consume starch, but this can be difficult to commit to with a family, so compromise and try one portion at breakfast and one for lunch. And instead of biscuits or crackers for morning and afternoon tea, try some fruit, nuts or seeds as a substitute.

As for the last two ingredients of the magic formula – fruit and vegetables – these are virtually interchangeable. Try and eat some of the portions raw. The fruit can be eaten for breakfast or throughout the day. The vegie or salad portions could be taken as a salad sandwich for lunch, or with rice or meat for dinner. It's very easy to do once you have the 2–2–4–4 habit embedded in your mind. All those other foods that we like to add to our diet such as dairy foods, sauces, herbs, garlic and chocolates are merely condiments to be eaten in moderation, they are not food sources.

This habit is a guideline for you. If you deviate a little, it's not the end of the world. But over the next couple of days, I'd like you to keep track of what you eat and see how close to the formula you come. If you're way off track, start by consuming four fruit portions a day, then move on to four portions of vegetables the following week and so on, until the 2–2–4–4 habit becomes part of your life.

ACTION STEPS FOR THIS WEEK

1

Each day this week make a note of how much
fruit, vegetables, starch and protein you are eating.

2

Try to get the food groups in their correct
proportions: 2–2–4–4.

29

DO NOT INDULGE!

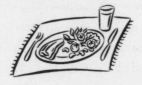

If you want to eat a lot, eat a little so you are around long
enough to eat a lot.

Tony Robbins

I remember watching the movie *The Meaning of Life* starring the Monty Python team. John Cleese played a restaurant waiter who was serving a very obese man. After serving him bucket loads of food, Cleese tempts the man to eat just one more morsel of food. After some persuasion, he eats a wafer-thin after-dinner mint . . . then explodes. It's meant to be funny, but as with most comedy, it is based on truth. Let's face it – we all have access to so much good food that sometimes we're not sure when to stop. And I'm sure there are times when you've eaten so much you've felt like you are about to explode.

Overeating is a habit. It may arise because you were

brought up during times of scarcity, and your parents insisted that you ate everything on your plate, or perhaps you just do it for comfort. I'm here to tell you that overeating is a habit, and it's a habit you can change. If you're an overeater, then now is the time to stop. The way I look at it, it's a question of control: does the food control you or do you control the food?

There are solid health reasons for stopping right now. Overeating causes health problems, shortens your life span, plays havoc with your digestion, encourages disease by making your immune system sluggish, causes a decrease in brain activity, makes you tired and lethargic, and can even lead to bulimia and other eating disorders. And you thought it just made you fat! I could go on and on about the bad effects of overeating but instead I'll give you some solutions to the problem.

Not long ago, I was listening to a very successful businessman and public speaker who admitted that one of the problems he had was overeating. It was one of the habits which was preventing him from achieving his goals. Then one day, he decided enough was enough! He was finally disgusted with himself (and when disgust sets in, that's the perfect time to change). But instead of handling the problem conservatively, he decided that the only way to break his habit was to attack it flamboyantly!

This man took a strong stance. He decided that when he found himself overeating, regardless of whether he was at home, at a friend's place or at a restaurant, he would throw down his knife and fork, jump up out of his chair, point to the chair, and in his loudest voice yell 'Pig, pig, pig!' Needless to say, it successfully broke the pattern of overeating and he changed his habits. Mind you, I'm sure there are a few restaurants where he is no longer welcome!

That's a pretty outrageous way of going about it. If you don't want to be so conspicuous, I'm sure you'll find a way to interrupt your overeating and break that habit. You'll feel much better for it. Usually when someone overeats, they feel very full and uncomfortable. If you overeat at dinner, you can wake up the next day with what I call a food hangover – feeling slow, befuddled and with a stomach in turmoil. Is it all worth it? That time you waste feeling horrible will never be returned. Life is too short to waste!

Whatever you do, don't expect a miracle cure for overeating. Creating a new habit takes time. You'll do well for a while, but there will be setbacks, moments when your old habits reappear. So pat yourself on the back for the times you do well, and get back on track as soon as possible if you slip up. Keep at it, and a new habit will form: refusing to overeat.

P.S. Now that you know what to do, re-read this chapter. Read again what overeating does to your body and make an informed decision then and there about whether you want to continue the habit of eating too much. Just remember who is in control – the food or you? Do it!

ACTION STEPS FOR THIS WEEK

1

Make a decision *now* and commit to changing your overeating habit.

2

Find an outrageous solution to stop you overeating, e.g. the 'Pig!' solution.

3

Do it!

30

ACID AND ALKALINE FOODS – AN EASY BALANCE

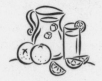

A wise person alters their life by altering their attitude.
Become the most positive person you know.

By this stage, if you have started changing your eating habits then you're probably already doing the habit change we're about to discuss without even thinking about it. So this chapter will be a good check to make sure all is going well and to give you some more information so that you know the benefits of taking this approach.

This chapter is all about acid and alkaline foods. What do those terms mean? Well, every food has both acid and alkaline elements. A food is termed acid or alkaline by the reaction it has on the body, and the end products left after digestion when all the particles of the food are turned into an acid or alkaline ash. This ash is what's left over after the body has used the food as an energy source. The minerals within a food are the main controllers of the acid–alkaline balance. The major acid minerals are: phosphorus, sulphur, silicon, chlorine, fluorine and iodine. The main alkaline minerals include potassium, sodium, calcium, magnesium, iron and manganese. The pituitary gland within the brain is the body's control centre for the acid–alkaline balance.

Alkalinity is essential for reproduction. An alkaline body promotes good health and energy, whereas an acid body is associated with ill health and lowered immunity. The body needs to be in an alkaline state to be strong and healthy.

I've heard many people say they can't eat a particular type of fruit 'because it's too acid'. But despite being an acid-tasting food, most fruits actually help to create an alkaline state, which is good for you.

Knowing all this, it makes sense to eat plenty of alkaline-forming foods and less acid-forming foods. But sadly, most western world diets are very acidic, contributing to the constant ill-health of colds, sore throats, infections and so on.

In previous chapters we've discussed foods which strengthen the immune system. And no surprises, alkaline foods are also great for your immunity. The chart on the following page shows you which foods cause the body to tend towards an alkaline state and those which lead to an acid state. When the ideal ratio is maintained, your body has a strong resistance to disease.

Alkaline Foods	Acid Foods
Most fresh fruits	Dried fruits
Most fresh vegetables	White asparagus
Sprouted legumes	Artichokes, brussels sprouts
Sprouted seeds	Legumes, pulses
Millet, buckwheat	Seeds, nuts
Rice	Wheat, rye, barley, oats, maize
Raw milk	Manipulated dairy products
Live plain yoghurt	Meat, fish, poultry
Herbal teas	Tea, coffee, soft drinks, alcohol
Chocolate	Drugs, food additives
Most fresh fruit juices	Packaged fruit juices

Food is not the only factor in creating a healthy alkaline environment in your body. Did you know that a person who is angry, unhappy, negative, selfish or jealous will build up an acid state in their body? Alternatively, a happy, positive, cheery, giving person will without doubt have an alkaline balance. We have the choice to react to a particular situation either in a positive (alkaline forming) way or in a negative (acid forming) way. Only you can make the decision; nobody forces it on you. For example someone may cut you off in traffic. You can either swear and curse at them and get mad, or you can let it go and realise perhaps they're in a hurry or perhaps they didn't see you. It is up to you.

A person who is in an acid state can expect more tooth decay, liver problems, a sluggish circulation, constipation, morning headaches, excessive mucus and even cancer. The increase in mucus production is because mucus acts as a buffer against the acid, so your body tries to cope with its acid state by producing more. Because most people tend to eat so many acid foods, excess alkalinity is very rare.

Balance is the key. The best ratio is four to one. That is, for every four alkaline-forming foods you eat, you should be consuming at least one acid-forming food. This is pretty easy to achieve. For instance, any of the breakfast recipes I suggested in the first chapter will give you a more alkaline start to the day.

For lunch, perhaps you'll have a salad-packed sandwich – once again, you're on the right track. And dinner, a piece of fish with four vegetables or salad. See – it's not that hard.

Some people need to pay even more attention to their acid–alkaline balance: heavy exercisers, women and professional sports people. This is because during strenuous anaerobic exercise, your muscles produce lactic acid. This acid has to be converted into another substance, or it will upset the acid–alkaline balance in the muscle, which can weaken it. In order to convert this lactic acid, vital enzymes and co-enzymes (minerals) are needed. Without these catalysts the lactic acid accumulates, resulting in stiff and sore muscles. Eventually (if the diet is sufficiently abused) permanent injuries and weakened muscles can be the result.

I hope you can now see how important it is to eat a correct balance of acid and alkaline-forming foods, no matter who you are. The right balance ensures vigorous health and energy. And that's what we all want!

ACTION STEPS FOR THIS WEEK

1

Be aware at each meal of the alkaline–acid balance.

2

Your diet should be 75 per cent alkaline, mainly fruits, vegetables and rice.

3

Only 25 per cent should be acid, mainly grains and proteins.

31

MICROWAVES –
TO USE OR NOT TO USE?

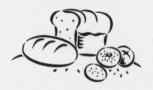

*It has become appallingly obvious that our technology
has exceeded our humanity.*
ALBERT EINSTEIN

Modern technology has changed the world our grand-parents knew. We have so many things in our lives that save time: washing machines, dishwashers, cars, ovens, microwaves, and the list goes on.

If all these time-saving devices are in use, why is it that everyone is so busy, and we don't have time to stop and chat, or help out a friend? People are so busy that they accept information as fact and don't question the authorities on matters such as technology, safe fuels, safe foods and safe medicines.

The use of microwaves and their safety is one area where complacency reigns. I have never felt good about microwaves, although I have used them on occasion with trepidation. I'd heard rumours of the dangers of microwave ovens but it wasn't until I read the research that I knew my instincts were right. I hope some of this information will make you think twice about using your microwave.

In general, people believe that microwave ovens don't have a negative effect on them or the food they cook. Of course, if microwave ovens were really harmful, our authorities and government would never allow them on the market, would they?

Microwaves are a form of electromagnetic energy, like light waves or radio waves. In our modern world, microwaves are used to relay long-distance telephone signals, television programs and computer information across the earth or to and from satellites in space. But microwaves are most familiar to us as a way of cooking food.

Every microwave oven contains a magnetron, a tube in which electrons (particles of matter) are affected by magnetic and electric fields, producing micro-wavelength radiation. This microwave radiation interacts with the molecules in food.

All wave energy changes polarity from positive to negative with each wave cycle. In microwaves, these polarity changes occur millions of times every second. As the microwaves generated from the magnetron bombard the food, they cause the molecules to rotate at the same frequency.

Put simply, all this agitation creates molecular 'friction', which heats up the food. This unusual type of heating also causes substantial damage to the surrounding molecules, often tearing them apart or forcefully deforming them.

Let's look at the some of the damaging evidence regarding the microwave oven.

Heating a baby's bottle in a microwave can cause slight changes in the milk and the loss of some vitamins in infant formulas. In expressed breast milk, some protective properties may be destroyed. Microwaving baby formulas converts certain trans-amino acids into their synthetic cis-isomers, which in plain English means that it makes the amino acids biologically inactive and therefore unavailable to the body. Furthermore, the amino acid proline is converted into a poison that is toxic to the baby's nervous system and kidneys. It's bad enough that many babies are not breast-fed, but now they are given man-made milk (baby formula) made even more toxic by microwaving.

In 1991, there was a lawsuit in the US concerning the hospital use of a microwave oven to warm blood needed in a transfusion. The case involved a hip-surgery patient who died from a simple blood transfusion. It seems the nurse had warmed the blood in a microwave oven which altered the blood and killed the patient.

Food scientist Dr Hans Hertel, along with Dr Bernard Blanc, studied the effects of food heated in a microwave on blood components of individuals. Significant changes were discovered in the blood samples. There was a decrease in all haemoglobin and a change in cholesterol values, especially the ratio of HDL (high density lipids) and LDL (low density lipids). Lymphocytes (part of the immune system) showed a distinct short-term decrease. In other words, heating food with a microwave oven compromises the immune system.

Dr Hertel was so vocal about this experiment that in 1993 there was a gag order put on him by the association of microwave oven manufacturers to stop him revealing more information about the dangers of microwaves. The gag order was lifted in 1998.

Put simply, microwaves change food.

By using plastic in a microwave you compound the negative effects of microwave-cooked food with toxins leached from the plastic, including phthalates (zeno-estrogens), which exhibit hormone-like behaviour.

I may be old-fashioned in my thoughts on diet and technology, but it seems that in the long run those old-fashioned actions may just be the saving of human health. Now that you have this information, it is up to you to change your microwave habit.

ACTION STEPS FOR THIS WEEK

1

Use the microwave oven less and less.

2

Cook your food by traditional methods.

3

Remember, just because you can't see it doesn't mean the danger isn't there.

32

FOOD
IN THE RAW

*The helping hands you are going to need in life are
located at the end of your arms.*
BRYCE COURTENAY

Most fruits and vegetables can be eaten raw, so why do we insist on cooking them to death and destroying the goodness in them? I believe it's simply a habit. Therefore this week's habit change is to see how many more foods you can eat raw.

There's no doubt about the advantages of raw food when compared to cooked food. Raw foods have an abundance of vitamins, minerals and, most importantly, enzymes. As we've discussed before, enzymes are the components of foods which help in the digestion process. Eating raw foods reduces the chance of overeating, increases health and vitality, and can reduce the chance of life-threatening conditions including heart disease, cancer and diabetes.

Cooked foods on the other hand have lost some of their vitamins, minerals and enzymes through exposure to heat, water and air. The longer food is cooked, the greater the loss of nutrients. Without the help of enzymes, some cooked foods take longer to digest and have a much higher chance of fermenting or putrefying in your stomach. On top of all that, the extra effort your tummy has to put into digesting cooked foods leaves you less energy to expend on the fun things in life!

Way back in the fifties, an experiment was carried out to see if eating raw foods made a difference to health and vitality. Two groups of people were chosen. The first group ate only raw foods; the second group ate only cooked foods. The results? The raw food group reported increased energy levels, said they were thinking more clearly, sleeping less, and generally had never felt so good. In contrast, the group which ate cooked foods felt no different, with some of them even feeling worse. I suggest you try your own experiment along these lines. For one week eat nothing but raw foods, and feel the difference. You will.

Another raw food experiment was conducted on milk, using five groups of mice as the subjects. Two of the groups were controls, one group was fed raw milk, another group drank homogenised pasteurised milk, and the final group was on sweetened condensed milk. The results were stunning.

By measuring coat texture, muscle texture and pathological lesions, the study established that the mice given raw milk had better health all round than any other group. What was more surprising was that the raw milk mice had increased vascularity to all muscle groups, whilst the other two groups had decreased muscle vascularity. The more vascularity you have, the faster oxygen and nutrients can reach your muscles. So if you're an athlete or someone just trying to get fit, raw milk can give you an edge. If only we could buy it.

Of course, not all foods can be consumed raw; some have to be cooked. But that doesn't mean we should cook every drop of food value out of them. Beware of anything which says 'ultra pasteurised' (like some fruit juices and long-life milks) as these foods and drinks have been heated, which could destroy some heat-sensitive nutrients.

In most states of Australia it is illegal to buy raw milk, which is a great pity. But it's perfectly legal to consume raw fruits and vegetables – or fish for that matter. The Japanese have a fabulous diet with a large amount of raw foods, and raw fish is a delicacy I highly recommend.

Foods which are best cooked for maximum digestibility include legumes (such as lentils, chickpeas, red kidney beans) and grains (whole wheat, millet, rye, oats). You'll find some recipes later in this book to show you how to cook these. Macrobiotic cooking methods are great ways to cook these two food groups for maximum nutrition and health. Another way to eat legumes and grains is to sprout them. This makes them easy to digest and increases the content of vitamins, minerals and enzymes.

Tomatoes are also a food enhanced by the cooking process. Tomato paste, cooked tomatoes, tomato sauce and the like have nutrients like lycopenes (powerful antioxidants) that are more readily available to the body than from raw tomatoes.

Cooking does not improve the value of food, although many would argue that it tastes better. The taste is just a matter of what you are accustomed to, so start eating some raw foods now. In the morning, instead of canned or stewed fruit, try grated pear or apple. At lunch, have a salad sandwich instead of meat or cheese. At night, have some salad with your dinner. And instead of reaching into the pantry for some crunchy potato chips as a snack, try a crunchy apple or pear instead.

Nature has provided an abundance of foods that we can eat raw – fruits, vegetables, nuts, seeds, some fish, sprouted grains and sprouted legumes. I'm not suggesting you only eat raw foods, but at least increase the amount you're eating now. I believe around 50 to 60 per cent of your diet should be raw foods, but it's up to you. Just remember, the more raw foods you eat, the more energy you'll have.

ACTION STEPS FOR THIS WEEK

1

Write down your diet over the next few days and see what percentage of raw foods you eat.

2

Increase the amount of raw foods you eat by having more salads and eating more fruit.

33

THE DRY FACTS
ON DRIED FRUIT

Sometimes things don't turn out the way they should.
If you have faith, you just need to trust that every
outcome is always to your advantage. You might not
know it till sometime later.

Dried fruit seems to be a popular snack food for young children, and some adults. It conjures up the image of a healthy alternative to sweets. You'll find piles of dried fruits in the health food stores, and from that we assume that it's a healthy food. But is it?

The history of dried food goes back to our hunter-gatherer ancestors. When fresh foods were abundant, our ancestors would dry their excess food so that they had something to eat when the winter months came and food was scarce. The food was usually reconstituted with water before it was eaten.

With food so abundant these days, we don't need to use dried fruit as a survival food source, but we consume it as a convenient snack. This is OK if it's done occasionally, but some people are eating dried fruit up to six times a day. For example, breakfast might be sultana bran or muesli, then some fruitcake for morning tea. Lunch might be a few slices of raisin toast, followed by some dried apricots in the afternoon and a dessert of plum pudding at night. Perhaps that's a little exaggerated, but I often see well-meaning parents give their children dried fruit constantly throughout the day.

Dried fruit is very hard to digest. Any parent who's been confronted by a nappy full of blown-up sultanas can attest to that! For these foods to be properly digested and assimilated by our bodies, it's important to add water. If water isn't added before you eat dried fruit, then your body has to add the water when the fruit reaches your stomach. This can dehydrate the body, and means by the time the dried fruit has become a real food again, it's already on its way out of your body before it can do any good.

Unless you're only going to eat a very small amount of dried fruit, I suggest you quickly boil it then leave it to soak in the water overnight.

Isn't it frustrating when you think you've been doing the right thing by eating a healthy alternative, and then I go and ruin it? Sorry, but wait till I tell you what they add to your dried fruit – it'll blow your socks off!

There are several things added to dried fruit, either during the drying process or after, and they're not necessarily on the food label. They are (get ready!) sugar, dextrose, glucose syrup, fruit juice, colouring derived from fruit, glycerin (422), sorbic acid (200), sulphur dioxide (220), paraffin, edible fats, and oils. Oil is sometimes marked on the ingredients. By the way, a quick way to tell if oil has been added is to look for a shiny, greasy appearance to the dried fruit. If oil hasn't been added, it will look dusty. And if oil is there, you can be sure that BHA (320) is also there. Good dried fruit (with nothing added) looks vastly different from the stuff you see on the supermarket shelves. Some of the effects these additives can have on humans include headaches, thirst, nausea, high blood sugar levels, skin irritations and irritations of the digestive tract, to name just a few.

So what's the alternative? Try to buy organic, naturally dried fruit. Or, dry your own. Food dehydrators are easy to find. Or on a hot dry day you can cut some fruit up thinly, place it on a metal tray or sheet, and dry it in the sun. Or you can pop the fruit into a convection oven on a very low heat for three hours or so. But remember that (even with natural, healthy dried fruit) it shouldn't be a constant food source. Eat your dried fruit occasionally and in moderation.

ACTION STEPS FOR THIS WEEK

1

Choose dried fruit that has been naturally dried – you will know by the colour.

2

Try to find organic dried fruit.

3

Remember, dried fruit is a treat – not a food source.

34

LET'S EAT
CHOCOLATE!

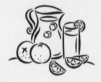

Winners are dreamers who won't give up.

For most of us, this change of habit is going to be a tough one – especially for the confirmed chocoholics. But don't despair, the news isn't all bad.

I have heard some people say that they crave chocolate so badly that they must have some every day. There are many theories that attempt to explain the craving for chocolate, with some people believing that it's caused by a mineral deficiency. But if that's the case, why don't we crave other mineral-rich foods like carrots? My theory on why some people crave chocolate is this: it tastes sooooooo good!

Here's the good news. Chocolate itself is not a bad food – in fact, it has some great food qualities. But there are two problems with chocolate. The first is the additives some chocolates contain. The second problem is how much of it we can consume in one sitting. So, avoid these problems and chocolate can stay on your shopping list. I can hear the cheering from here!

When it comes to chocolates, most people seem to find that their willpower totally deserts them. So this chapter is about how to rid yourself of chocolate cravings, yet still get to eat some. To accomplish that aim, there are a few ground rules to follow.

Rule #1

Eat only the best chocolate, made from the finest ingredients. I choose home-made chocolates or European ones. More often than not, these have fewer additives and chemicals. The main ingredients that you are looking for are cocoa, cocoa butter, organic cane juice (rapadura sugar) and milk.

The reason?

Once you've got a taste for these delicious chocolates, chances are you won't be willing to settle for less.

Rule #2

Only buy single, individually wrapped chocolates. No family blocks, no assorted boxes, just one!

The reason?

Firstly, they're so expensive you won't want to buy too many. Secondly, they're not available at every store like common chocolate, and they taste so good you're not likely to put up with a not-so-nice chocolate.

Rule #3

When you get that one chocolate in your mouth, savour it, enjoy the experience, and make it last.

The reason?

Because that's all you get!

Rule #4

If Rule #3 fails and you want another chocolate, that's OK, but you must return to the same store and buy one single chocolate again.

The reason?

If you keep returning to buy a single chocolate time after time, the shop attendant will think you're a nutcase. The strange looks they give you might make you stop and think.

Rule # 5

Stay away from all other chocolates for the first two months of this change.

The reason?

We don't want you regressing.

It might sound like I'm the one who's becoming a nutcase, but trust me – it works. Once you're accustomed to the fabulous taste of high-quality chocolates made the old-fashioned way, that huge family block will seem less appealing. You'll find yourself doing without if you can't have the best. The change will take time, but soon you'll be wondering when the last time you had chocolate was. It sneaks up on you gradually. Like this entire healthy living plan, you just do it bit by bit, and all of a sudden you realise that a lot has changed.

Now, let's talk about the other chocolate products in the grocery store – chocolate drinks and chocolate sauces. I recommend you take a close look at the food labels on them when you do your shopping this week. Decide for yourself whether you're willing to keep swallowing them. Once you read the labels, I believe you'll think twice. If you do want a chocolate drink, then buy organic cocoa, whole milk and rapadura sugar and enjoy it on occasion, with no excess additives like colours and flavours.

Today is the day you start your new approach to chocolate. So, when you're in the corner store and all those yummy chocolates start calling you, look for that little individually wrapped high-quality chocolate that tastes great. And if it's not there, walk out.

Good luck. I promise the next habit change will be an easy one!

ACTION STEP FOR THIS WEEK

1

Find out where you can buy high-quality chocolate. Have a taste and never look back.

2

Follow the chocolate rules strictly for at least eight weeks without deviating. It works!

35

HOW SWEET
IT IS

*I learnt more from my failures than I ever did from
my successes.*

BRADLEY HARRIS WOLF (AGED 14)

After all these chapters, I am just now getting to the topic
of sugar. Don't panic – it's not as bad as you think, at least
when sugar is compared to all the other sweet rubbish out
there.

We have been eating sugar and honey for ages. It's only
since our obsession with calories began that sugar has become
the big bad ogre. It's time to set things straight.

First, let's talk about the alternatives – the artificial rubbish.
Artificial sweeteners such as saccharin and cyclamates cannot
be metabolised or used by the body, which is why they have nil
calorie and kilojoule values. Aspartame is a different case – it is

200 times sweeter than sugar, so much less is used, and we therefore take in fewer calories.

Saccharin was banned in the USA, but was returned to the market after a huge public outcry, despite the health risks that caused its withdrawal in the first place (including links to bladder cancer). Yep, you get just one calorie, but what else is it giving you?

In 1981, the US Food & Drug Administration approved aspartame (Nutra-sweet®). By 1985, the American Medical Association believed it was safe and so it was promoted as a product for a healthy lifestyle which did not have any cancer risks, unlike cyclamates. But what we weren't told is that once aspartame is in the human body, it changes into aspartic acid, phenylalanine (an amino acid) and methanol. Increased levels of phenylalanine in the body have been associated with poor muscular co-ordination and may adversely affect the brain and nervous system of those people who can't metabolise phenylalanine properly. (These people are identified at birth and put on special diets.) Methanol is a particularly poisonous alcohol.

There are reports that women who have consumed aspartame during pregnancy have an increased chance of having a child with brain damage, and that children who are fed aspartame in the first six months of life may possibly have a higher chance of incurring brain damage. In adults, aspartame can cause headaches, inappropriate behaviour responses and seizures. It has also been linked to brain tumours. Not very appealing is it! Have you heard enough? There is plenty more, but I won't go into the details.

What I can't understand is why we are even considering

these 'foods' as alternatives, when the effects won't be known for years or even generations. I can tell you I won't be taking any chances with them and I don't intend to be part of some giant human experiment – so I choose not to eat technology-based or artificial sweeteners.

The trend seems to be to find a sugar with no energy value. As each year passes a new one is created. Be aware that each one promises much but may deliver more sinister conse-quences than just one calorie.

Corn syrup, otherwise known as high fructose corn syrup (HFCS), is found in many packaged and prepared foods. There are many studies that show this is a sweetener to avoid as much as possible.

The complicated process for making HFCS out of corn was developed in the 1970s. There are three different enzymes, two of them genetically modified, required to break down the cornstarch, which is made up of chains of glucose molecules of almost infinite length. It is broken down into the simple sugars glucose and fructose – mostly fructose, hence the name. Con-ventional wisdom is that fructose is better for diabetics than sugar, but every cell in the body can metabolise glucose, while all fructose must be metabolised in the liver. Studies show the livers of rats on a high-fructose diet look like the livers of alco-holics: cirrhotic and fatty. Not only does it affect the liver, but studies have also shown an increase in colorectal cancer in women associated with diets high in HFCS, and there is a growing number of studies that point to HFCS being a major player in the obesity epidemic.

Since studies have revealed that the effects of high fructose are most severe in the growing body, it's important to think carefully about what kind of sweeteners are fed to children. Fruit juices and cordials made with corn syrup should be strictly avoided, as they are very high in fructose, and so should anything with HFCS, such as jams, condiments, sauces, muesli bars and soft drinks. HFCS is also a favourite in many health food items, so read your labels.

There are other sugar syrup alternatives that are found in our food supply, like glucose syrup, maltose and fructose to name a few. They sound natural, but they come from foods that have been tampered with and had ingredients added. Glucose is never found by itself in nature – it's always linked with fructose. There's a good reason for that: glucose enters the bloodstream very quickly, giving you a fast energy boost, with the fructose following behind to maintain your energy levels. Without fructose, the glucose has no backup. You'll fall flat on your face with no energy once the glucose is used up. The combination of glucose and fructose is found in sugar and honey in the right harmony.

So why don't manufacturers just use sugar? I believe there are two reasons – because sugar has become a dirty word, and because man-made syrups are often up to 40 per cent cheaper than sugar itself, making profitability higher for the manufacturer.

So what do you use if you have a sweet tooth? The best you can do is go back to the natural stuff – honey, pure maple syrup, pure organic raw sugar, molasses, fruit and all those natural things. There's enough there to satisfy the sweetest sweet tooth. Of course, some of these products are processed, so be very picky and buy the best quality you can.

You'll notice that I haven't included sugar in the natural list. The common thought is that the best sugar to eat is organic raw sugar, but it goes through many processes. It begins with juicing of the cane, then the syrup is heated, lime, canola oil and icing sugar are added, and then there is more processing. At the end of the first processing stage, raw sugar is the result. This sugar is then sent to a refinery, where it goes through many more steps before it becomes pure white sucrose, with no nutritional value whatsoever. So why eat a food totally devoid of nutrition when you can eat a yummy sugar with loads of nutrition? The best is sugar cane juice that has been simply dehydrated. It not only tastes good but has most of the nutrition from the sugar cane. This sugar, called rapadura, is not found in many supermarkets, but can be sourced from health food stores and organic food outlets. You will also find it in many health products such as organic chocolate and other delicious foods.

Always remember to read the food labels on any sweet foods to see what they're using to sweeten it.

ACTION STEPS FOR THIS WEEK

1

Throw away any foods or drinks that have artificial sweeteners.

2

Be aware of sugar syrups, especially high fructose corn syrup or corn syrup in packaged foods.

3

Go back to natural sweeteners – honey, maple syrup, palm sugar and rapadura (see Appendix for supplier).

4

Enjoy all sweets in moderation.

36

SUGAR
FOR HEALTH

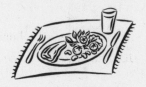

*Technology . . . is a queer thing. It brings you
great gifts with one hand, and it stabs you in the back
with the other.*

C.P. SNOW

Emerging technologies are changing the way we live our
lives. Of the top ten newly emerging technologies around
the world, three have to do with the human body and our
health. These are not the latest you-beaut machines to save
lives – they are completely new technologies that will trans-
form medicine and health.

One is the emerging technology of glycomics. This is the field
of understanding and ultimately harnessing sugar. Why would
anyone want to harness sugar? The latest research reveals that
sugar can be converted into a drug to tame the immune system

and minimise damage following heart attacks and surgery, as well as other drugs that could have an impact on health problems ranging from rheumatoid arthritis to the spread of cancer cells.

Sugar is a nasty word to the health-conscious, but I guarantee that as more information comes to light, sugar will soon be the new health buzz word.

Let's look at the field of glyconutrients, or the science of sugar nutrition. The first myth about sugar is that all the sugars the body needs can be manufactured from simple glucose. It is now known that this is not the case – cells prefer to utilise non-glucose essential sugars. The second myth is that sugar is nothing more than a fuel needed for energy. Research is uncovering that this is not correct – sugars are necessary for far more than energy.

The health effects of vitamin and/or mineral deficiency are common knowledge, as is the fact that the wrong types of fats can cause disease. Since sugars are found on every cell in every organ of the body, it should stand to reason that some sugars are also vital for proper function of the body and that without them health problems can emerge.

Over the last few decades researchers have slowly uncovered clues to sugar function. Of the more than 200 known sugars, scientists have discovered that eight are essential for optimal function of the body. They are xylose, fucose (not to be confused with fructose, the fruit sugar), glucose, galactose, mannose, n-acetylglucosamine, n-acetylgalactosamine and n-acetylneuraminic acid.

You've heard about essential fats and amino acids (protein) – now there are essential sugars (carbohydrates). All three macronutrients have essential components. These sugars are *absolutely essential* to glycosylation: the adding of sugar to the protein on the cell membrane, to help with cell communication. These sugars coat each and every cell in the body. They are now known to be the actual communicators between cells, not proteins as was once thought. This cellular communication system is known as 'multicellular intelligence', determining which nutrients and substances are needed for the health and wellbeing of a particular cell and its function. In other words, without these communicators there can be no organised life.

If cells do not have the right sugars, they are unable to send the right messages about their needs. For instance, essential sugars are very important in establishing blood types – O, A, B and AB. They can literally determine life or death, not only for each individual cell, but eventually for the organ for which it is responsible.

The body can, in theory, produce the other seven essential sugars from glucose, but it is a long, energy-draining process. If there are any enzyme, genetic, metabolic, disease, free radical, toxic load or other problems in the body, the sugars are not created properly or in enough quantities, and the person will eventually become sick.

Sugars also help the brain and nervous system – from memory and sleep to anxiety and depression. In addition, they have a role in helping the body control cholesterol and fats by lowering triglycerides and low-density lipoproteins (LDL) while, at the same time, raising the high-density lipoproteins (HDL).

Another important function of essential sugars is to help retain bone density and muscle mass. The body undergoes wear and tear as it ages. Cells and tissues need to be replaced, remodelled and renewed continually. Exercise helps the body to develop new blood vessels while increasing muscle mass. Certain kinds of tissues adapt to exercise by increasing the size and number of cells. Adaptation, healing and recovery are all forms of tissue remodelling. Essential sugars play important roles in these processes.

As I mentioned, scientists theorised that all glycoprotein sugars were constructed from the glucose we eat. This theory stood for many years without testing. Recently, however, new technology has proven this glucose-only theory to be false. We now know that the body not only absorbs these various essential sugars intact from the gastrointestinal tract, but, in many cases, prefers to obtain them from our diet. Obtaining these sugars from dietary sources is more efficient than obtaining them through multi-step enzymatic conversions from glucose because less energy and time is required.

So if you want optimal health long-term, it is essential to eat the right foods with the right sugars in them. Following is a table that lists the eight sugars and their food sources.

Food Sources of the Eight Essential Sugars

Essential Sugar	Food Source
Xylose	Guava, pears, blackberries, loganberries, raspberries, aloe vera gel, kelp, echinacea, psyllium, broccoli, spinach, eggplant, peas, green beans, okra, cabbage and corn

Fucose	Medicinal mushrooms, seaweeds, kelp, wakame, brown seaweed and brewers yeast.
Glucose	There is obviously no shortage of glucose in the average diet, but the following provide some better sources of dietary glucose: honey, grapes, bananas, cherries, strawberries, mangoes, cocoa, aloe vera, liquorice herb, sarsaparilla herb, hawthorn, garlic, kelp, echinacea, rapadura and sucanat.
Galactose	Dairy products, most fruits (but highest in mangoes, plums, rhubarb, prunes, oranges, nectarines, peaches and blackberries), echinacea, fenugreek, chestnuts, and most vegetables (but highest in carrots, brussel sprouts, leeks, asparagus, pumpkins, parsnips, cauliflowers, onions and cabbages).
Mannose	Black or red currants, gooseberries, green beans, capsicum (cayenne pepper), cabbage, aloe vera gel, fenugreek, guar gum, eggplant, tomatoes, turnips, shiitake mushrooms and kelp.
N-acetylgalactosamine	Bovine (gelatine) and shark cartilage (shark cartilage should not be used by diabetics or those with kidney disease).
N-acetylglucosamine	Bovine and shark cartilage (see note above) and shiitake mushrooms.

N-acetylneuraminic acid (sialic acid)	Whey protein, hen eggs and other animal and human substances.

The first time I was introduced to the science of sugar nutrition was when my sister-in-law told me she gave her old dog glucosamine tablets for his arthritis and it helped. Glucosamine, a derivative of n-acetylglucosamine, is a very popular natural remedy for osteoarthritis in humans. Mannose is now sold as a remedy for urinary tract infections. Xylitol and mannitol, the sugar alcohols of xylose and mannose respectively, are now sold as sugar in health food stores. Without us even knowing, these essential sugars are being introduced into our daily lives. Make it a point to learn about them and to introduce them into your diet.

Studies have shown numerous benefits of the eight essential sugars, ranging from increased immunity on all fronts (including antiviral, antibacterial and antiparasitic), to accelerated wound healing (especially burns), reduction of allergies and slowing of the aging process.

It all seems too good to be true, but I look at this in perspective. The body is an amazing machine; we do not know everything about it. Every time I read research, especially newly emerging research, I realise that the full complexity of the body is far beyond the reaches of science as we know it today. The wisdom of the body is far-reaching – it knows what to do and it knows how to be healthy, but it needs the right fuel. Glyconutrient research is just another field that tells me that natural foods are the best to eat, not technology-driven or processed foods. Check through the list of foods that contain the eight essential sugars, add them to your diet and make sure you eat them on a regular basis.

We need to trust in the body's ability to do the right thing. The research is great but the bottom line still says the same thing: nature has provided the food that the body needs for health. The manipulation of food by technology, creating the foods which now line our supermarket shelves, is an abomination to the intelligence of the human body.

ACTION STEPS FOR THIS WEEK

1

Start eating foods with the essential sugars.

2

Check through the list of foods and make sure you are eating at least one from each essential sugar.

3

Enjoy the benefits of better cell-to-cell communication.

37

ALCOHOL –
IT'S A SOCIAL CHOICE

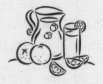

Most of our diseases are brought upon ourselves by
smoking, bad diet and overuse of alcohol, caffeine
and soft drinks.
DERRICK LONSDALE MD

Consuming alcohol is a choice. Some religions direct and some people choose to abstain, while others enjoy the occasional glass of wine with their meal. And then there are the Saturday night binges.

Alcohol has a long history. Beer is thought to have emerged around 4000 BC. Wine came into prominence around 3000 BC. These drinks have been used for religious ceremonies, for their medicinal properties, and for the pure joy of it! They are certainly widely used.

There is evidence that alcohol can have a protective action

against heart disease. It may also protect against cancer. There have been many studies made throughout the world which support this. A recent study in Germany supported the theory that moderate beer drinkers have a reduced risk of heart disease and other illnesses – 'moderate' being a glass a day. This will not work if you save up all your 'one glasses' for that Saturday night binge.

What I have told you are the good things about alcohol, but it must also be pointed out that while it helps the circulatory system it also has detrimental effects on health, even in moderation. It depletes vitamin and mineral stores which, in turn, affects all the systems in the body. Alcohol also overloads the liver. The liver must break it down into its components so that the body can either use it or expel it.

Alcohol is very soluble. In fact, even in the mouth, alcohol is absorbed straight into the bloodstream. Once in the stomach it is rapidly absorbed, so much so that if you drink on an empty stomach at least 90 per cent of the alcohol will be absorbed within the hour. Alcohol clumps the blood cells together causing the blood to thicken, slowing down the flow of oxygen to the brain. The thick blood leads to blockage of the blood flow through some of the brain cells. When the oxygen supply is cut off completely, brain cells die within three to twenty minutes. In short, by the time your social drink makes you feel happy, you have already begun to kill off brain cells. A heavy drinking binge could damage as many as 100 000 brain cells. Worse news is that this damage is permanent. Brain cells do not reproduce and cannot be replaced.

Alcohol is not a stimulant, but a narcotic. For some people, a glass of beer impairs intelligence and weakens memory. The smallest dose will impair judgement and reasoning. The bad news continues, because alcohol in small doses decreases immunity and – guess what! – it slows down your metabolism.

The latest research shows that alcohol is dangerous for the unborn child and should be strictly avoided during pregnancy. A study took place over 25 years examining the risk of alcohol disorders on children. It found that young adults whose mothers drank as little as three glasses of alcohol on any one occasion in the early stages of pregnancy were more then twice as likely to develop an alcohol problem. It is well established that alcohol exposure during pregnancy can affect the structure and function of a developing foetus, interfere with the development of the central nervous system and cause a range of disabilities.

So if you weigh up the bad and the good, I would say the scale is very weighted on the bad side. So now that you know all the facts, think again before you have that daily glass of alcohol.

If you still choose to drink alcohol, once again choose the best. During the processing and manufacturing of wine, beer and spirits, additives are used – some for the advancement or balance of the process, some for preservation of the product. Sulphur dioxide (220) is used universally in both beer and wine. There are some wine manufacturers who are now not adding (220), although during fermentation some sulphur dioxide is produced, but only a small amount. If you are an asthmatic or have gastrointestinal problems, liver or kidney malfunction, then I suggest that if you want to drink wine, you choose one without preservative added. There is also a growing number of wine growers that are now choosing organic methods, so more and more organic wines without preservatives are becoming available.

With any alcoholic beverages, choose the best; choose those made traditionally. But for total health I believe that what researchers call moderation is still too much. An occasional social drink would be far better for long-term health, along with a good supportive diet.

As for spirits, these are almost always drunk with mixers. Most mixers such as cola, lemonade and ginger ale are where the problems lay, as these drinks have an uncanny way of leaching calcium stores out of your system. They are definitely not healthy. If you must have the occasional bourbon or rum, then try it with water or straight – like the good ol' days. The mixers will always be your downfall, including the diet ones.

ACTION STEPS FOR THIS WEEK

1

If you are a daily consumer of alcohol, try cutting down your consumption and have some alcohol-free days.

2

Check the additives in your wines and choose one with fewer additives.

3

Consume spirits straight.

38

ELIMINATE
CHEMICAL CALORIES

The system of nature, of which man is a part, tends to be
self-balancing, self-adjusting, self-cleansing. Not so with
technology.

E.F. SCHUMACHER

As you've probably figured out by now, I'm not one to count calories. Having said that, I believe that we need to start a new practice – counting our chemical calories; that is, the amount of chemicals we take in on a daily basis.

The body's in-built intelligence for natural weight and health is being compromised and we are being poisoned by the array of toxic chemicals that we encounter in our everyday lives – many we unknowingly use or consume without any realisation of what they are doing to the body. This damage makes it increasingly difficult for our bodies to control weight and maintain health, so we are getting fatter and sicker, even though we may be eating less food, less fat and exercising more.

The body's basic desire is homeostasis. It is constantly adjusting to make sure our temperature is correct and mineral balance, both in and out of cells, is maintained (this is so you don't retain water and blow up like a balloon, or not have enough water and look like a prune). The body maintains a toxic-free environment by taking the good stuff from what we consume by way of eating, breathing and skin absorption, and excreting the rubbish through urine, faeces, carbon dioxide and sweat.

The body also has some tricks up its sleeve. If it can't eliminate all the waste due to an overload, and cannot maintain homeostasis, it packs waste away where it can't do damage until given the opportunity to get rid of it. Some people, in their whole life, never give the body that chance and thus create a neverland of waste throughout the body. So where is this neverland? You guessed it: the fat cells often called cellulite! Toxic synthetic chemicals used in agriculture, skin care, cosmetics and household products are highly fat-soluble. The more toxic you are, the more fat your body will lay down to protect itself from the toxins.

If the body becomes overloaded with toxins it will initiate a severe elimination process – a so-called cold or flu. The toxins are dumped into the mucus and the body will excrete as much as it needs to in order to maintain some sort of order. But, more often than not, people hate colds and the associated mucus, so they take medications to stop the flow of mucus and thus the elimination of toxins. This compounds the problem, creating fatter, less healthy individuals and, eventually, more severe colds.

But wait – it gets worse. There is another group of synthetic chemicals that have been contributing to the obesity rate in different way. They are termed carbamates. This group of insecticides and herbicides used on our fruits and vegetables, and as an ingredient in cosmetics and medicinal preparations, is also used as a growth promoter in battery-farm chickens because they slow down the metabolic rate. So the same synthetic chemicals used on our fruit and vegetables are used to fatten livestock! Not surprisingly, carbamates are also used in medicine to promote weight gain in humans. You have to wonder where the logic is in that. One way of improving your metabolic rate is to not eat foods that have been sprayed with carbamates – in other words, choose organic.

I've never believed that one thing alone – such as calorie counting, cutting out fats, increasing protein, reducing carbohydrates, eating only grapefruit or eliminating chemicals from your diet – is the answer to the obesity and health problem. But what I do believe is that it is a change in lifestyle that will make a difference, and every positive step along the way will take you to your goal. This habit is about decreasing your chemical calories.

So how do we do this? The first step is food. By now you should know what to do, but to reiterate: eat only good, wholesome, nature-based, organic (if possible) foods.

The second step is looking at what you put on your skin. The skin is the largest organ we have. It absorbs and eliminates, so anything you put onto your skin will make its way into your body. The same rules apply here as they do for food. Go to your bathroom right now or before the day ends and read the ingredients on your shampoo, conditioner, moisturiser, lipstick, toothpaste, etc. You'll be astounded by the list of chemicals whose names are unknown to you. A great rule of thumb for cosmetics is: if you can't eat it, don't put it on your skin. It's really exciting that there is a groundswell of people who are now making cosmetics and skincare from organic food ingredients. By hunting these down and using them you will eliminate another large amount of chemical calories.

The third step to eliminating chemical calories is to take a good, hard look at your household cleaners and detergents. These products are minefields of toxic chemicals, and although you don't use them on your skin or consume them, you do inhale them. Any contact with these chemicals can create an increase in chemical calories and thus an increase in ill health and obesity and a decrease in energy. For many years I used vinegar, bicarbonate of soda and ammonia for cleaning, until I was introduced to a line of cleaning cloths made from special fibres. The cloths work better, using only water – what an easy way to decrease your chemical calorie load.

In case you're not sure whether making this lifestyle change will work for you, let me tell you about someone I know. My friend is an avid exerciser and has been since her youth. Despite an active lifestyle, she had been 14 kg overweight for many years and she'd had enough. After discussing chemical calories with me she decided to eliminate the chemicals in her life. She threw away chemical household cleaners, and her entire makeup and skincare collection, and replaced them all with natural organic products. She also started buying organic foods and eliminated all foods labelled low-calorie or low-fat. What is amazing about her diet is that she didn't necessarily change what she was eating, she simply made sure her food was organic and whole. Over a twelve-month period she managed to lose all the excess weight. Changing this habit changed her life – it can change yours too.

You are never going to eliminate all the toxic chemical calories in your life, but you can cut them right down so that your body has a chance to eliminate the load, rid itself of excess fat and create health and more energy.

ACTION STEPS FOR THIS WEEK

1

Check out all the products in your bathroom and follow this good rule of thumb – if you can't eat it or pronounce it, don't put it on your skin.

2

Proceed to your laundry and check your cleaning products. If a poison caution is included anywhere on the label, then throw it out and look for non-poisonous products or specialist cleaning cloths.

3

Buy organic food as much as possible.

39

SUNBATHE EVERY DAY

The best six doctors anywhere, and no-one can deny it,
are sunshine, water, rest, air, exercise and diet.

WAYNE FIELDS

Choices are what determine attitude. You can choose to have a happy disposition or to be downright unhappy. The choices you make are often determined by the way you feel, both physically and mentally. In order to make good choices it is important to do everything in your power to maintain health. Eat nature-based foods, exercise (incidentally and with planning), take time out for relaxation, and enjoy health-giving sunlight every day.

Without sunlight we would be dead. The sun has been given some bad press over the past 20 years, which has created a fear about exposure. Most people won't go out into the sun without sunscreen or sunglasses, many completely covering every limb and body part with clothes. We need sunlight every day.

The sun has the ability to block the hormone melatonin from being produced in the body. Melatonin is the sleep hormone and when your skin is exposed to direct sunlight it ceases to be produced, thus awakening the mind and senses for an energetic day. Then at night when the sun goes down, melatonin is produced again, getting you ready for sleep.

Sunlight and outdoor living are the best ways to obtain vitamin D, a fat-soluble vitamin that is stored in the body for a very short period of time. Vitamin D regulates all vitamin and mineral metabolism, especially that of the minerals calcium and phosphorus. It controls calcium levels in the body to help in the prevention of osteoporosis. It is also essential for the function of the brain and nervous system, as well as the performance of muscles. Vitamin D is important for the growth, maintenance and repair of all bones and teeth. Together, it's a daunting task for a single vitamin.

In the far reaches of the northern hemisphere, some people who have very little natural sunlight exposure are diagnosed with SAD (Seasonal Affective Disorder), also called winter depression or winter blues. This disease is characterised as depression due to lack of sunlight. The further away from the equator you live, the greater the likelihood of this disorder. Sufferers endure oversleeping but without the feeling of refreshment, as well as overeating, depression, irritability, lethargy and lowered resistance to infection. Women, children and adolescents seem to be most vulnerable to this condition.

Seasonal Affective Disorder is due to a lack of bright sunlight. Researchers have proved that bright light makes a difference to the brain chemistry. This disorder is not an imaginary illness. The cure is exposure to sunlight (or a specially designed light), every day.

But wait a minute! Here I am telling you how wonderful sunlight is and that you should expose yourself as much as possible, yet for the past twenty years you've been warned of the dangers of the sun, especially in relation to ageing and cancer; more specifically, melanomas. Sunlight is not the menace. It is far more complicated than that. Melanomas are not caused by exposure to the sun. After all, if the sun was the cause of melanomas, everyone who went out into the sun would get a melanoma, and this is definitely not the case. As I've said, with any disease, lifestyle is the determinant. It's not usually one thing that causes a disease but a combination of factors. So let's explore some of these factors.

Diet, of course, is one of the most important factors. Everything you put into your mouth becomes the re-building blocks for your body. Put good stuff in and the results will be good; put bad stuff in and the results will be ill health and early aging.

Processed and refined foods, lacking many vitamins, especially B6, increase the skin's sensitivity to light. The fat we consume changes the composition of the fat beneath the skin's surface, once again increasing the skin's sensitivity to light – beware of manipulated man-made fats such as hydrogenated vegetable oils and margarine. Some prescription medication (antihypertensives, tranquillisers, hormonal drugs and antibiotics) can change the tolerance of the skin to sunlight. Artificial sweeteners are also added to this list. In fact, hundreds of chemicals have been documented as photosensitising agents (agents that cause the skin to react to light differently).

An increased number of adverse skin reactions were reported after the introduction of fluorescent light in the 1930s. In 1941, a study found that dermatitis was caused by prolonged exposure to fluorescent light. Then in the '70s and '80s, other studies revealed that exposure to fluorescent light at work doubled the risk of melanoma. There is increasing evidence of higher incidences of melanoma among indoor workers and, even more astounding, the melanomas appear on body parts least exposed to sunlight.

The fact is that natural light differs from all artificial light in the intensity of the light wave, the colour spectrum, distribution and aspects of filtering. Consider also other factors that may change conditions of natural light, such as the use of sunscreens or even the type of clothing worn. It is interesting to note that when the use of nylon stockings became prevalent in society there was also an increase in lower limb tumours in females. Nylon stockings were suspected of changing the quality of natural light on the skin.

Sunlight is very important for health, wellbeing and survival, but many people abuse the sun. During the week these people spend their days indoors working in an office under artificial light, and then spend the weekend as sun worshippers, without any regard for its power. Wearing sunscreen stops the burning ultraviolet rays but there are two other ultraviolet rays that can cause damage to the skin in other ways.

Most sunscreens don't stop these rays. The burning of the skin is a good indicator that you have had enough sun. This is the body's wisdom taking care, but sunscreens mask that indicator and people tend to stay out in the sun too long.

To ensure a healthy amount of sunlight, spend time outdoors every day before ten and after three, avoiding as much as possible the hottest period of the day. If you need to be out in the hottest time of the day, wear a hat and shirt and make sure you choose 'natural' sunscreen with the least amount of chemicals possible.

More importantly, make sure that you have the immunity to fight off the dangers of skin cancer. Eat natural and wholesome foods to ensure the building blocks of your skin are at their healthiest.

ACTION STEPS FOR THIS WEEK

1

Look for a 'natural' sunscreen.

2

Wear a hat and shirt in the midday sun.

3

Sun your skin every day (before ten and after three).

40

HOW TO NEVER TAKE
ANOTHER ANTIBIOTIC

If your GP or paediatrician often prescribes antibiotics
for colds and flu, then I have one piece of advice:
find another doctor.
PETER J. D'ADAMO

If you want to get off antibiotics here's where to start. Eating right is the first step towards staying healthy. But if for some reason you feel like you're coming down with a cold, or just feeling run down, your diet can be an integral part of getting well without having to resort to the use of antibiotics and medication.

Let me explain how. First, let me tell you about myself, because I believe I'm living proof of how this can work. Many people tell me I am lucky with my health, but I can tell you that luck has nothing to do with it. Taking responsibility for your own health, and taking the initiative to get well and stay well is what it's all about.

I am forty-six, and I have never had an antibiotic. I have never taken paracetamol or an aspirin. I have never been immunised. I've told many people about this, and they are absolutely amazed. What surprises me is that I've never met another person who can say the same. My children are 13, 15 and 17 and they have never had any medications either, including antibiotics. They get fevers but I allow them to run their course, and they get colds so we change their lifestyle and get them to slow down. If children don't learn to fight the little ills in their childhood by themselves without intervention from medication, then how are they to fight the big ills as they get older? Of course, there are points where medication is needed, but for the most part the body is very clever in healing itself of childhood ills. We just have to give it the right foods so that the immune system is working at top gear.

I think that perhaps I was destined for this healthy lifestyle, and to teach it. Back in the forties, my grandfather was a farmer in Iowa, USA. When pesticides and chemical fertilisers were introduced, my grandfather refused to use them. He believed they would be the downfall of traditional farming. Of course, he was ignored or laughed at, but, in hindsight, he was way ahead of his time.

My grandmother also remained 'old-fashioned' with her cooking, baking her own breads and preparing and canning foods from my grandfather's organic fruit and vegetable garden.

My mother followed in their footsteps by always feeding the family only the most natural of foods simply prepared. As a chiropractor, my father was very much into preventive health. He refused to have his children immunised or give any medication, unless in a life-threatening situation, as he was uncertain of the ramifications.

So, there's a potted family history, which probably explains why I tend towards the natural. Hey, I figure, I'm still alive at forty-six, and with more energy than most people that age or younger, so I must be doing something right! If you choose this way to health, you'll be surprised at how easy and effortless it actually is.

My son was hurt in a football accident at the age of 13. We realised very quickly that he had probably broken his collar bone. The X-ray at the hospital confirmed a clean break and the broken bone virtually looked like a lopsided cross. A nurse asked my son what his pain was like, asking him to give the pain a number between one and ten, where one wasn't bad and ten was very painful. My son said eight. Immediately the nurse said that she would give him an injection to help him with the pain. Without any prompting from my husband or me, my son told the nurse he didn't need it. I knew at that point that the way my husband and I had taught our children and brought them up had been tested and our methods had worked. My son made it through the entire break and healing process without any form of medication or pain-killer. It was his choice.

A friend of mine recently called me and asked what she should do for her 14-month-old son who was grizzly with a new tooth coming through. I told her to allow him to experience the pain, and let his body create the endorphins that help him cope with pain. Most mothers give a pain-killer to their children whenever they have an ache or pain. This stops the body's natural pain-killers from taking action, and as the saying goes, if you don't use it you'll lose it. If you don't give the body the chance to develop its own pain endorphins when dealing with the small pains, then they are never going to work with the big pains. My parents did this for me, and I do this for my children. Parents who follow my method see the difference.

For most people, great health doesn't require antibiotics and medications. When you are not well with a minor ailment, you need to look at your lifestyle rather than running to your GP for another pill to pop. I'm always amazed at the number of people who head for the doctors when they've got a cold, and are carelessly prescribed antibiotics. The common cold and some other ailments are just the body's way of saying, 'Stop – give me a break! Start looking after yourself, eating more fruit and vegies, and give me a chance to fight this bug!'

I believe we depend too heavily on medications to get us well, rather than pursuing a healthy lifestyle with an emphasis on nutrition. Many mainstream doctors are becoming aware of this. We now know that ear infections are the most common reason for antibiotic use among children, with 15 million prescriptions written annually in the US. Antibiotic resistance is a growing, worldwide public health concern that has been spurred by the widespread overuse of the drugs. In many developed countries, approximately 96 percent of doctors treat ear infections immediately with antibiotics, even though most cases will resolve on their own without treatment.

There are foods which can boost your immune system, and

others which drain your immunity. By now I'm sure you can guess what those foods are.

Immunity boosters are fresh fruits and vegetables, and cooked grains such as rice or barley. Good old-fashioned barley and vegetable soup with lots of garlic is one of the best ways I know of combating a cold. Immunity-draining foods are all processed foods, from cereals and breads to fats and dairy foods, without exception.

So when you're feeling not-quite-right, start by having fruit for breakfast, rice salad for lunch, and barley or vegetable soup for dinner. And drink plenty of pure fresh water. After twenty-four hours, you'll start feeling a lot better, but don't go back to immunity-draining foods just yet. You need to stay on this regime for a period of three days, so that your body has a chance to fight and eradicate the virus or bacteria which is causing your illness. On top of that, you need to rest, as rest helps the body to heal.

It's that simple! Your body starts to fight its own battles again without relying on outside help from antibiotics or other medications. The old saying 'If you don't use it, you'll lose it' also goes for your immune system. If you allow antibiotics to fight your fights, then one day your immune system will just pack it in and not know what to do, as is the case with auto-immune diseases.

So next time you feel an illness coming on, try it my way. It's a great sense of achievement to overcome the adversity just by looking after yourself. Let the body's own immune system look after you, rather than letting a bottle of tablets strip you of your natural immunity.

ACTION STEPS FOR THIS WEEK

1

Take responsibility for your own health.

2

If feeling a little unwell, change your diet.

3

For strong immunity eat fruits, vegetables and whole grains simply prepared.

41

ORGANIC –
WHAT'S THE POINT?

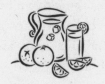

The saddest aspect of life right now is that science gathers knowledge faster than society gathers wisdom.
ISAAC ASIMOV

The use of chemicals on farms in both animal husbandry and crop production has created environmental and human health disasters. Many chemicals that were introduced during the 1950s are now banned due to their link with cancer and other diseases, yet we continue to make new chemicals and farm with them without knowing the full ramifications of their long-term effects. Time will tell!

Many people ask me about the need for organic foods, although today, with up to 75 000 chemicals floating around the environment, it is hard to get truly pure chemical-free, organic foods. Despite this, I still insist that there is a need to buy as much organic produce as you can afford. Why continually bombard the body with more and more chemicals? I'm not just talking about organic fruit and vegetables, but also meat, flour, grains, sugar, dairy, cereal and the like. These are all available in grocery stores, selected butchers and many health food stores.

The benefits of eating organic food are far-reaching. Not only does the body benefit, but so does the environment and all the animals that live on this planet. When you choose foods that have been produced by sustainable agriculture you are helping so much more than just your body. As consumers we are all powerful. If we choose to buy organic foods, it increases the demand, which, in turn, leads to more farmers using organic practices, and that has to be good for everyone and everything. The more people choose these foods, the cheaper they will become.

Organic foods have higher levels of vitamins and minerals. A recent study conducted by the Australian Government Analytical Laboratories, comparing vegetables grown in biologically revitalised soils with conventionally grown vegetables, found that, on average, the organic group was ten times higher in minerals such as calcium, potassium, magnesium, sodium, iron and zinc.

Many people in western society are showing signs of chemical saturation. This is a condition where the body is bombarded over many years with a progressive assault of chemicals, through food and water, air pollution, chemicals in skin care, indiscriminate use of medications, and many other avenues. Up to a point, the body shows no signs and then one day a small amount of chemical from some source triggers an illness that is unexplained, with symptoms including tiredness, headaches, persistent colds, skin irritations and a generally unwell feeling. As long as you continue to bombard the body with chemicals then the symptoms will persist. More often than not, these collective symptoms are termed chronic fatigue syndrome, a disease that did not exist just 25 years ago. Conventional medicine offers no cause or cure, but I can guarantee that a body in this condition can take no more.

In order to be a vigilant consumer with regard to organic foods, it is important to know what you are buying. The Australian Quarantine and Inspection Service (AQIS) is the sole government regulator of organic agriculture, production and processing, and is responsible for enforcing standards and legislation for exports. AQIS has approved seven organic grower organisations that monitor their member producers to ensure they adhere to AQIS standards, and while most of their produce is exported some remains to be sold in Australia. If the seal of approval from these regulatory bodies is not on the food then you must trust the person selling you the produce, because in Australia there is no regulation for the use of the term 'organic'.

AQIS standards for organics include that all fruit and vegetables must be cultivated free of pesticides in soil fed with animal and plant waste. Livestock must graze on organic pastures and the use of growth hormones or chemical treatments is forbidden. Intensive housing of animals is banned, as are long periods of artificial light. Farms must be sustainable to ensure the future health of the land.

The food you put into your body will determine its health. Eating organic does not mean eating only bean sprouts and lentils. You can eat any food you want, from chocolate cake to homemade lemonade – whether they are healthy or not is all about the ingredients you put into these foods.

Many people say, 'It's all too hard and too expensive!' As I've said before (and I believe it is worth repeating): the effort and money you put into your health in your youth will ensure that the effort and money you put into sickness and ill health later on in life is minimal. And believe me, there are many people who suffer debilitating diseases that last half a lifetime or longer. Two out of three Australians will suffer a life-threatening disease. My mission in life is to be the one who doesn't. Make it your mission too.

ACTION STEPS FOR THIS WEEK

1

Find an organic supplier in your area (see Appendix).

2

Become aware of the symbols for certified organic food, which can be viewed at www.changinghabits.com.au, and the names of the certified bodies, which appear in the Appendix.

3

Begin to include organic foods in your diet.

42

POTS, PANS
AND PACKAGING

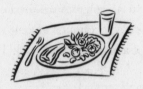

*Excellent health is based on natural principles. It grows
over time with proper nutrition, regular exercise, rest
and a great attitude.*

A healthy diet isn't just about food, it's also about the utensils you use to cook and store the food. It's one of those things most of us would never think of, so that's what this chapter is all about – making you more aware.

Research has shown that aluminium cooking pots and utensils can be a health hazard. If you've owned aluminium pots and pans for a long time, you might have noticed them getting thinner over the years. The reason for this is that the aluminium is slowly wearing off, leaching into the foods you cook. This is dangerous because aluminium is inorganic.

So what's the difference between organic and inorganic

minerals? Inorganic minerals come from the ground (rocks, soil etc). During photosynthesis, plants take up these inorganic minerals from the ground and convert them to organic minerals, which our bodies can easily assimilate and use. I guess that's why we don't eat rocks and soil for dinner!

Our bodies can absorb inorganic aluminium, but it forms residues, especially within the arteries. It can have a weakening effect on the entire digestive tract and damage the efficiency of vitamins in the body. Excessive aluminium levels have been linked to Alzheimer's disease and dementia, which is becoming increasingly common amongst the elderly.

Other sources of aluminium you should be aware of are baking powder, some white flours, vaccinations, children's aspirins, antiperspirants and even false teeth. Symptoms of aluminium toxicity to watch out for include constipation, nausea, skin problems, lack of appetite, profuse perspiration, cramps and lack of energy.

Cast iron pans are another one to watch out for. Once again, the iron coming off the pan is inorganic. Our bodies cannot use this form of iron. In fact, it will chelate (join) with other minerals and elements, rendering them useless to the body.

I would also stay clear of coated, non-stick pans unless you buy a very good product and take extremely good care of them by using the right utensils and not overheating them. Inferior products, over a period of time, can lose their coating due to wear and tear by scraping. And where does that coating go? Into your mouth. Now unless you have a hankering for the taste of non-stick coatings, why would you eat them?

After 50 years of non-stick coating use, evidence is mounting that one of the key ingredients, perfluorooctanoic acid

(PFOA), stays in the environment indefinitely and can be found in the blood samples of children and adults. Another chemical found in the fumes of non-stick coatings is polytetrafluoroethylene, (PTFE), which was discovered in 1941. The danger of PTFE is that the fumes are odourless and colourless, and it is not clear how long it lingers in the air.

In 1951, the first case of a human suffering from PTFE problems was reported. Polytetrafluoroethylene produces flu-like symptoms and is called 'polymer fume fever', but it's rarely fatal. For birds, contact with PTFE fumes can often prove fatal, sometimes within as little as five minutes of exposure.

It's worth being aware of these chemicals and their possible problems so that you can make informed decisions about whether you want to continue using a product.

Just about every household has plastic storage containers. You've probably eaten food that has been stored in plastic and noticed a peculiar taste and smell to it. This makes me wary of plastic containers. I had a client who spent fifteen years working in the plastics industry. With his knowledge of plastics, he refused to have plastic food containers in his home, and will not eat foods which have been stored in them. It makes you wonder what he knows!

More research is coming to light that various plastics, such as the polycarbonates found in baby bottles and water jugs, have the ability to mimic natural oestrogen. These mimics (termed zeno oestrogen) are highly fat soluble and non-biodegradable. They have a tendency to accumulate in the fat tissue of animals and humans and are very difficult to excrete. There are many hormone mimics, and up to fifty have been identified. The effects worldwide on humans, animals and plants range from reduced sperm production to interference with growth and development, changed behaviour responses, decreased intelligence and reproductive problems. So where possible, reduce the use of plastics.

So how about plastic wraps? Did you know that they contain an additive which is not permitted in foods intended for infants and young children? That's because the plastic has a chemical on its surface which has been known to increase cholesterol levels in the blood, and break down the Vitamin D in our bodies. You can live without plastic food wrap. I've done so for the last two years, and after a short while, you don't even miss it.

So which food storage utensils are the best to use? Glass, stainless steel and crockery are the best. These three materials do not leach anything into foods that are prepared and stored in them.

Changing from plastic containers to glass, and trading in your aluminium pots and pans for those made of stainless steel or glass can sometimes be daunting, but if you make the change slowly over time, it's not that difficult.

And while we're on food containers, let's talk packaging. All food seems to be surrounded by packaging – plastic, aluminium, styrofoam and cardboard. When you start changing your habits and eating more wholefoods, you'll notice your weekly rubbish is dramatically reduced. Some weeks after recycling I only have one small bucket of rubbish to go into the wheelie bin, for a family of five.

To reduce packaging even more, purchase the bags that are now sold at many grocery and corner stores and take them when you go grocery shopping. They hold more and don't break like plastic bags, and using them reduces the number of plastic bags you accumulate. When I go shopping for things other than food, I take a calico shopping bag with me. Yes, you're only one person doing it, but it does make a difference.

ACTION STEPS FOR THIS WEEK

1

Try to reduce the number of plastic bags you use when shopping.

2

Throw away any coated cookware that has chipped.

3

Think of ways to stop or reduce the use of plastics.

43

BEWARE
IMMORTAL FOODS

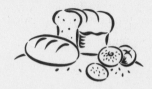

The work of an individual is the spark that moves
mankind forward. This is the power of one.

The dictionary defines immortal as *not subject to death* or *imperishable*. Imperishable is the word which should grab your attention. Any food which does not perish should immediately be suspect. You should be asking yourself *why* it won't perish.

Let's compare a mortal food (like a fresh apple) with an immortal food (like a famous-brand hamburger). If you left both of these foods on a shelf for four months, what do you think would happen to them?

After four months, the famous-name hamburger would still be there, perhaps looking slightly shrivelled. The apple would be gone, with perhaps just a few pips left. I remember discussing this during a presentation I gave to about eighty people, and one lady simply wouldn't believe me. 'What about the buns?' she asked. I suggested that if she didn't believe me, she should try an experiment for herself. If you have doubts, try it for yourself. The buns will still be there four months later.

Why is this so? Well, food goes off. When the micro-organisms in the air land on a mortal food, they love it. They start eating the food, and they thrive and multiply till all the food is gone, as you've no doubt seen. When these same micro-organisms land on a food with little nutritional value (like the famous hamburger) they die. That's right – they die; so there-fore the food never spoils.

Our bodies are made up of cells which are very similar to those micro-organisms, except we're a lot more complex. So the way I see it, it should take a lot more of those famous-name hamburgers to kill us, but also a lot more fresh apples to make us healthy and energetic.

Some of the foods your family is eating may well be immor-tal. If you're not sure, test them by placing them on a shelf for a while to see what happens to them. Here are just a few foods you might like to try: chocolate, cheese-flavour baked snacks, chips, highly processed takeaway foods, processed cheese (especially cheese slices), soft drinks, fruit drinks, candy, processed meats and some cereals. The cheese slices are really interesting. My kids and I tried the experiment using pro-cessed cheese slices, and they ended up looking and feeling like slabs of plastic.

It's no great surprise that these foods will last forever. After all, many of them contain high levels of preservatives, and these chemicals are simply doing their job – preserving something, almost indefinitely.

Of course, the nutritional value of a food isn't the only factor which affects the working of micro-organisms, but it's an important one, and gives you some understanding of what immortal foods are all about. After all, put bad stuff in and you'll get bad results, or put good stuff in and you'll get great results.

Now let's talk about *mortal* foods. Fresh fruits and vegies are right at the top of the list. Also fresh meat, chicken, fish and biodynamic raw milk are mortal foods, as they quickly spoil. Then there's a group of foods which are suspended in time by nature's own preservative. Foods like nuts, whole grains, seeds and eggs, all encased in the natural packaging of their own shell. No artificial preservatives required.

So, when you're trying to work out if a particular food is a healthy choice, as well as asking yourself, 'Is this food close to its original source?', you should also ask, 'Is this food mortal?' If the answer to both questions is yes, then go for it!

ACTION STEPS FOR THIS WEEK

1

When you eat a food, think!

2

Ask yourself: is the food you are about to put in your mouth mortal (nutritious) or immortal (no nutrition).

44

CHEATING IS A PART
OF THIS DIET

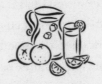

The way you describe your day becomes your day.
Always answer a greeting with 'excellent' and see
what happens.

What is a diet without a bit of cheating? The fact is that most people cheat on their diets, so why not incorporate that cheating into your diet plan, and then you won't feel so guilty. That's what this week's habit is about – eating what you want for approximately three meals a week. Or, better still, living by the 80/20 rule: 80 per cent of the time, eat healthy food where you know what it's made of, and 20 per cent of the time take a break.

Being deprived of your favourite foods can be hell on any diet. But with a diet for life (like this one), the thought of no luxury foods *ever* can really turn people off.

There has been so much research and publicity on diets and nutrition that we're all tired of hearing 'Eat less fat, salt and sugar'. So why are people eating so much of these three foods? The reason is that these three ingredients are the ones that make food taste so good! I must admit that when it comes to deciding what to eat, it's difficult for nutritional advice to compete with the pleasurable sensory experience of eating some foods.

Just the right amount of fat, salt or sugar added to a food is called the bliss point. This is the point at which fat, sugar or salt is added to a particular food at just the right level to evoke maximum pleasure when eaten. If the wrong amount of these ingredients (too much or too little) is added, the experience can be worse than no sensation at all – like your favourite soup with way too much salt. Food manufacturers are masters at using the bliss point principle. They work hard to make sure their processed foods hit your bliss point, to make sure you go back and buy more.

For most people, the drive to eat is a chase for this pleasurable experience. People say they are eating less salt, fat and sugar, but the paradox is that as a nation Australians are consuming more of these commodities, and as a consequence we're getting fatter and less healthy.

So why do our heads tell us one thing, but our stomachs crave the opposite? For the answer, we have to go back a few thousand years. As we've discussed before, our ancestors primarily ate fruit. Fruit is at its nutritional best when it is sweet, so over time we evolved to like this level of sweetness, and to look for it. It's interesting to note that the sweetness bliss point today is still the level produced by a ripe orange, apple or pear – around 10 per cent sugar by the weight of the fruit. So it doesn't make much sense trying to totally eliminate sweet things from your diet when you're fighting thousands of years of evolution!

The love of salty things is also etched into our genes. Just as we do for sugar, we have specific taste buds on our tongue for salt. Salt stimulates the tactile receptors in your mouth, firing into action other sensory channels and boosting the overall impact of those sensations when eating. You'll probably be surprised to learn that our primary source of salt isn't junk food, but grain products such as cereals and breads. Eating bread that contains no salt is a bit like eating cotton wool – a bland experience.

So, if you want to eat the right things, your willpower will need to be pretty strong, because you're fighting your genetic makeup. So how do you cheat without blowing your whole diet? The key is to cheat in moderation. I suggest a maximum of three 'cheat' meals a week, which allow you to reach your bliss point in either fat, sugar or salt. This should keep you satisfied. But don't forget ripe fruit will also keep your sweet bliss point satisfied. Nuts and avocados will satisfy the fat bliss point and by adding sea salt to your grains (rice, oats etc) you can keep the salt bliss point happy too.

A diet entirely made up of healthy wholefoods will ensure you a long, healthy life. But a diet with mostly healthy foods plus a few splurges every now and then ensures you a fairly long, healthy and happy life! Live the 80/20 rule.

ACTION STEPS FOR THIS WEEK

1

Make sure eating is a pleasurable experience by having just the right amount of sweetness, saltiness or fat in your meals. Go to *your* bliss point.

2

Live by the 80/20 rule.

45

SUPPLEMENTATION – IT'S NOT WHAT IT SEEMS

*A new philosophy and a new way of living cannot be
achieved without effort. It is acquired with much
patience and effort.*

The vitamin and mineral industry is a big industry making
billions of dollars. It is not always about health but more
often about profit.

Over the last few decades there has been a plethora of
research on vitamins, minerals and other nutrients and what
good or bad things they do to the body. As a result people have
been self-prescribing and professionally prescribing supplements. There have been scares about overdosing and sure
signs of malnutrition, but who is to say what is right?

The usual scenario is that if you have an iron deficiency then
you take an iron supplement, if you have a calcium deficiency

then you take calcium. But that is not the way the body works. It is not a tit for tat system, it is much more complicated than that. Yet we seem to be treating it that way, and sometimes this can have serious consequences.

Let me give you an example. The buzzword around fifteen or so years ago was vitamin A. There was extensive research being conducted throughout the world showing how vitamin A was good for nearly any ailment. One particular research was done over a ten-year period on men. In the study there were two groups: one group took vitamin A every day and the other group took no vitamin A. The study was stopped after eight years as the researchers realised that the males taking the vitamin A were dying at a far greater rate of heart disease and cancer than the group not taking vitamin A. When I read this study I was perplexed at first, but then it dawned on me. Of course! Vitamin A, especially from a laboratory, by itself, is not how nature intended it: it must be with other food components or it can cause an imbalance in the body's chemistry, resulting in disease.

I always go back to the same old thing: what nature gave us is best. Nature does not give us a vitamin or mineral by itself but with other nutrients, which are synergistically bound together in a perfect mix – food! Nature knows everything. Man is just beginning to learn, and I do not believe that nature will give up all her secrets.

Mother Nature seems to give up her secrets very slowly, as is evident by the latest nutrient discoveries. In the last decade scientists have found nutrients in our foods called phyto-nutrients. They are like vitamins. It is believed that there are thousands of phytonutrients in our foods, yet we have only just recently discovered them. Therefore those so-called complete supplements that you were taking fifteen years ago, made in a chemical laboratory, did not have any phytonutrients. And who's to say that the supplements you take today are complete. The only supplement that can be complete is food.

There is always the argument that the food we eat today is inferior, compared to 100 years ago. And yes, I am the first to agree that most of our foods are devoid of many essential minerals because our soils are lacking. Our foods are stored for such extended periods of time that the vitamins and phyto-nutrients become next to nothing. The chemicals that are sprayed on our foods also affect their nutrient values. But let's look at the other side. These days most people aren't even eat-ing enough fruits, vegetable, grains and seeds, but are, instead, eating refined breakfast cereals, refined breads, refined fats and so on. I wonder if our nutrient deficiencies would be as great if we started eating normal foods again. Buy organic foods and eradicate the above problems.

If you are someone who does not eat well, then more than likely you will have nutrient deficiencies. Symptoms can be varied but the best one of all is 'munching'. When the body needs nutrients it will often make you want to eat. It is an inbuilt mechanism for survival. Animals also get this problem of munching. When the animals start chewing on rocks and fence posts then the farmer knows they have a mineral defi-ciency (called cribbing or pica) and they know the solution is to put a salt block with minerals in the paddock. The animals lick the salt block and the munching stops. Humans, well that's a different story; we don't munch on fence posts and rocks, we munch on non-nutrients, snacks such as chips and sweets, and we continue to do it, instead of seeing it as a sign of a deficiency and doing something constructive about it. The answer is to change those habits and start eating nutrient-filled foods.

Once the diet is in order then supplementation is just that: a supplement to a good diet, not a substitute because of a bad diet.

If you choose to supplement then here are some guidelines to help you choose an ethical and nature-based supplement. When choosing a supplement choose one from nature. For example a food or herb that has been organically grown on nutrient rich soils, dehydrated and concentrated and then put into a capsule or a bag to be sold. This will perhaps not have the high concentrations of laboratory-made supplements but will have the right balance. And remember, quality is better than quantity. What is wonderful is that this is where supplementation seems to be going. More and more companies are coming up with this idea, realizing that nature will give us the answers to health. Typically, for protein I won't buy a powder, I'll eat a raw egg. For fat, I buy cold-pressed oils, like flax, almond, avocado and the like. If I need minerals, I buy liquid colloidal minerals from ancient vegetable deposits. Vitamins and phytonutrients can be easily obtained from wheat grass juice or barley green. These are all foods rather than chemicals from a laboratory.

Reading labels of supplements is just as important as reading food labels. I remember looking at one popular brand of children's supplements and realising that perhaps it had an artificial sweetener within. The label said there was no cane sugar but failed to say there was no artificial sweetener. Immediately I was suspicious as I wondered how they made it sweet.

I rang the company and inquired about the sweetener. Yes, there was aspartame in the supplement. Aspartame is a man-made sweetener, a neurotoxin, which causes havoc within the body. You must read between the lines and grill the manufacturers until you are satisfied that what you are taking is a whole natural product without any dangerous additives.

It is very important to learn about the product, the ethics of the company and exactly what is put into the supplement. And if you think that is too much hard work then think again! This is your only body: know what you are putting into it and don't rely on someone else selling you a product that they believe is OK.

ACTION STEPS FOR THIS WEEK

1

Read the food labels of all the supplements you have in the house.

2

If you are unsure about any product call the manufacturers and ask for all ingredients.

3

Find out if the nutrients in supplements are from a laboratory or from food.

4

Throw out any that are suspect and find a supplement that is based on food.

46

PUTTING IT
ALL TOGETHER

Remember there are no failures;
only learning experiences.

If you have worked through each of the habit changes (and stuck to them) then by the time you reach this chapter there really shouldn't be too much to do. But let's put it all in perspective.

The way of eating I propose in this book is very easy and very simple. You don't need fancy recipes, and you don't need to weigh foods, check fat content or count calories. I have put a few of my favourite recipes in the back of this book, as well as in my *Changing Habits, Changing Lives Cookbook*, but there are many recipe books available and all you need to do is substitute natural foods for any poor-quality ingredients in a recipe. For instance, if margarine is used in a recipe then replace it with butter or cold pressed oil. If they suggest using skim milk powder and water, use diluted whole milk instead. If it says to use salt, make it sea salt. Replace white flour with organic unbleached flour, and so on. This diet enables you to use most of your existing recipe books – just make sure you're following the habit changes. The best rule of thumb when it comes to recipes is the K.I.S. principle – *keep it simple*. Exotic French dishes are a delicacy, whereas meat and salad with a vegetable is more likely the norm for this diet. It's really simple once you get into the swing of it. You'll find that most healthy meals are very easy to prepare, and the combinations of different foods are endless – as long as they are fresh and natural, not man-made or manipulated.

Remember, this is not a diet to achieve change overnight. Actually, in the strictest sense of the word, it's not really a diet at all: it's a way of life that should stay with you forever, not just the next two weeks. Once you experience this way of eating and living, you will never look back.

Whatever you do, do it at your own pace, not at anyone else's, because the right pace for one person will not suit someone else. You don't necessarily need to follow these chapters in any particular order, although I do recommend that you avoid starting with the Cheating chapter! The chapters are in the order of my recommendations, but you can be flexible. You will also find that many of these chapters overlap in some areas, but that's OK because it just makes each habit change that much easier.

Exercise is a valuable extension of this lifestyle. Throughout evolution humans have exercised, whether it was chasing the woolly mammoths for dinner, or working in fields to grow crops, or doing heavy physical work during the industrial revolution. It wasn't until the information age just forty years ago that things changed. Now we have machines and equipment to do most of our heavy labour, with the majority of us pushing paper across a desk or using a computer. This makes it imperative that exercise be incorporated into our weekly routines, making up for all that physical labour which we evolved to do. Exercise is important for bowel regularity, resetting the metabolism, increasing fitness, improving circulation and muscle tone, and many other aspects of your health.

If you've made it this far into this book, you'll have a pretty good idea of what you should be eating each day to suit your lifestyle and your likes and dislikes. If you're like me (with too much to do every twenty-four hours) then cooking isn't always practical. That's another advantage of this diet – it contains so many foods that you can eat raw. They're easy to obtain and simple to prepare. Fruit is my number one snack food, with fresh nuts and seeds following closely behind.

When it comes to keeping variety in your diet, I find that I stick to one breakfast day in, day out for a couple of weeks, then I change to a new breakfast. Others, like my mum, are religious about having a variety of breakfasts. She writes down a breakfast menu for each day of the week. But you don't have to do it that way – whatever suits you, please do. Your lunches and dinners also need to be varied, so make sure that each day you follow the 2–2–4–4 Magic Formula fairly closely – that will give you the variety you need.

Go back and review this book often, and when you find

yourself a bit off track, just start again. You'll find that many of the habits have remained and that you're probably only slipping up on a few of them. As time goes on, the habit changes will become part of your life and you won't entertain any other way of eating. Remember, this diet has stood the test of time. It has got us to this point in history and it can take us further, for I believe that a diet devoid of natural foods such as fruits, vegetables, nuts, seeds, fresh meat and grains would ensure our eventual extinction.

At my website, www.changinghabits.com.au, you can enjoy my monthly newsletter to stay informed about food and health. The more knowledge the better, and knowledge is a great motivator for change.

Whatever you do with these habit changes, make sure you have fun. Enrol a friend to make the changes with you so that you can spur each other on. And when it works for you, pass the book along so other people can benefit. There are too many people out there suffering because of lack of energy and health. And too many people with complexes about the state of their bodies, believing that they are either too fat or too thin.

By changing your lifestyle you can have the energy you need to do the things you *have* to do, and plenty left over to enjoy the things you *want* to do. Have fun!

47

MEAL PLANNING

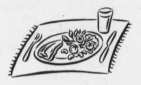

*Don't let a day go by without learning and trying
something new and interesting. A successful person
never stops learning and trying.*

These are just suggestions for you, but you can make up your own meals by following all the habit changes. You will notice that I have a menu plan for winter as well as for summer. If you feel you don't need a cheat meal then don't take it. I find if I do have a cheat meal and it has been a good cheat then for the following meal I usually just eat fruit or a salad.

Winter Menu

	Breakfast	Lunch	Dinner	Snacks
Monday	New Age Porridge	Cheat meal	Lamb roast and vegetables	a.m. fruit p.m. fruit
Tuesday	Meal on Toast	Baked bean jaffles	Vegetarian Spaghetti	a.m. fruit p.m. fruit
Wednesday	Cyndi's Muesli	Pumpkin soup with home made bread	Vegetable stew and rice	a.m. fruit p.m. fruit
Thursday	Rice Porridge	Vegetable soup and cornbread	Cheat meal	a.m. fruit p.m. fruit
Friday	Fruit Only	Salad sandwich on rye bread	Fish and vegetables	a.m. cheat snack p.m. fruit
Saturday	Red Date Congee	Eggs on toast	Lentil Burgers and salad	a.m. fruit p.m. fresh nuts
Sunday	Protein Shake	Barley soup	Roast chicken and vegetables	a.m. fruit p.m. cheat snack

Summer Menu

	Breakfast	Lunch	Dinner	Snacks
Monday	Fruit Only	Corn pasta and pesto with green salad	Chicken and salad with broccoli	a.m. fruit p.m. fruit
Tuesday	Cyndi's Muesli	Salad sandwich on rye bread	Quiche and salad	a.m. fruit p.m. fruit
Wednesday	Fruit Only	Green salad with pine nuts	Potatoes and salad with roasted cashews	a.m. fruit p.m. fresh nuts
Thursday	Meal on Toast	Cheat meal	Vegetarian Lasagne and salad	a.m. fruit p.m. fruit
Friday	Red Date Congee	Salad sandwich with wheat bread	Fish and beans and salad	a.m. fruit p.m. fruit
Saturday	Protein Shake	Eggs on toast with tomato	Cheat meal	a.m. fruit p.m. fruit
Sunday	Cheat meal	Salad with cornbread	Red meat with potatoes and salad	a.m. fruit p.m. fruit

RECIPES

I have incorporated just a few recipes that you may not have in your current recipe books. These are favourites of my family and I thought you may also enjoy them.

Vegetarian Lasagne
Part One
500 g good ricotta
1 organic free-range egg

Mix together.

Part Two
Fresh lasagne sheets

Part Three
1 tbsp oil
1 brown onion – chopped
3 cloves garlic – crushed
450 g pre-cooked whole brown lentils
750 g organic pasta sauce (spaghetti sauce)
1 cup filtered water

Heat the oil. Add garlic and onion and fry gently, then add the lentils and fry for one minute. Add the spaghetti sauce and water, mix and simmer for 20 minutes. Set aside.

In a large lasagne dish cover the bottom with part one mixture, then put a layer of part two, followed by a layer of part three. Repeat until all the ingredients are used, finishing with a layer of part one. Sprinkle some grated cheese on top and place in a 180°C oven for 20 minutes. Serve with a large green salad.

Vegetarian Spaghetti
1 pkt soba noodles (buckwheat)

Cook as directed on pack.

1 tbsp cold-pressed oil
3 cloves garlic – crushed
1 onion – chopped
450 g pre-cooked whole brown lentils
750 g organic pasta sauce (spaghetti sauce)
1 cup water

Heat the oil. Add garlic and onion and fry gently, then add the lentils and fry for one minute. Add the spaghetti sauce and water then mix and simmer for 20 minutes.

Potatoes for Dinner
1 large or 2 medium-size Pontiac potatoes per person

Steam potatoes until just cooked through (test with a fork).

Lettuce – shredded (adjust quantity to suit numbers)
1 avocado – diced
1 carrot – grated
1 large stick celery – sliced

1 red pepper (capsicum) – sliced or diced
Baked beans (organic) – 2 tbsp per person

Dice potatoes and put in a serving bowl. Add a couple of table-spoons of baked beans straight from the tin, cover with shredded lettuce and all other ingredients. Dress with garlic dressing (see below).

Garlic Dressing
6 cloves garlic – crushed
2 tbsp fresh herbs – chopped (whatever is in season)
2 tsp seeded mustard
1 tsp fresh ginger – grated
½ tsp sea salt
Pinch of black pepper
1 bay leaf – crushed
200 mL cold pressed olive oil
30 mL lemon juice

Place all ingredients in glass jar and shake. Keep refrigerated. If you want a more creamy dressing add 2 tbsp pure sour cream.

Meal in a Salad
1 head of fancy lettuce (Waldorf, Butter) – shredded
2 medium carrots – grated
¼ cup cheese – grated
½ red pepper (capsicum) – chopped
½ green pepper (capsicum) – chopped
1 avocado – chopped

1 tomato chopped

3 tbsp sunflower sprouts, or whatever sprouts you have in the fridge

2 sticks celery stuffed with macadamia nut butter – chopped into 1 cm pieces

¼ cup pine nuts roasted

2 tbsp gomasio (see below)

Gomasio

120 g roasted sesame seeds

10 g sea salt

Mix and crush. Keep in refrigerator, and use on steamed vegetables, salads, rice, or mixed in soups.

Hummus

450 g pre-cooked chickpeas

3 tbsp tahini

1 tbsp cold pressed olive oil

6 tbsp lemon juice

½ tsp salt

1 to 3 cloves garlic (at your option)

2 tbsp chopped coriander

Place all ingredients in a food processor and mill to a fine paste. Serve as a dip with rye crackers.

Potato Salad

Pontiac potatoes (1 large per person)

Cook potatoes. Allow to cool, cut into quadrants.

1 red pepper – chopped
2 tbsp organic sultanas
2 tbsp pine nuts – roasted
2 spring onions – finely chopped
1 tbsp gomasio
2 tbsp homemade mayonnaise

Cook potatoes and allow to cool. Mix all ingredients together in a serving bowl.

Cornbread

175 g yellow cornmeal
1½ tsp bicarbonate of soda
½ tsp sea salt
1 organic free-range egg
150 ml yoghurt
1 tbsp honey
2 tbsp cold pressed oil

Mix all dry ingredients (cornmeal, bicarb soda, sea salt) thoroughly; add all other ingredients and mix well.

Pour into a lightly greased loaf tin and bake at 200°C for 15 to 20 minutes. Turn out on rack and cool. Variations: if you want a sweeter loaf, add more honey and dried fruit; for a more savoury loaf, add chopped peppers, or onion with some paprika.

Lentil Burgers

225 g pre-cooked whole brown lentils – mashed

100 g fresh breadcrumbs or cooked rice

50 g fresh nuts – ground

100 g good (hard) cheese – grated

1 clove garlic – crushed

1 tsp marjoram

1 tsp basil

½ tsp sea salt

Pinch of freshly ground black pepper

Flour, seasoned (pinch sea salt, black pepper)

Combine all ingredients, chill for about an hour. Shape into burgers, and dip into egg and then into seasoned flour. Shallow fry for about 5 minutes on each side. Serve with a large green salad.

Rice Porridge

1 cup rolled rice

1 tbsp organic sultanas

1 tbsp organic dried bananas

2 cups water

½ tsp sea salt

Mix all ingredients, soak overnight.

Bring to the boil then simmer for 5 minutes or until porridge consistency is reached.

Serve with grated apple, yoghurt, and honey if desired.

Almond Nut Milk
1 tbsp raw almonds
1 cup warm water
Honey – optional

Blend until smooth. This is great for pouring on the Red Date
Congee or any of the other cereals. I use it in place of yoghurt.

Cashew Nut Butter
1 cup cashews
3 tbsp orange juice

Blend together until smooth. Use more orange juice if needed
or, for a more creamy nut butter, use olive oil in place of
orange juice. You can use any nut for a nut butter. Experiment
with different ones.

APPENDIX OF
ORGANIC SUPPLIERS

If you are not sure where to get organic fruit, vegetables, meats, herbs, nuts, seeds and eggs you may call any of the following groups and they will put you in touch with someone in your area. If they are not able to help you, call your local health food store.

Following is a list of stores certified by the National Association for Sustainable Agriculture, Australia (NASAA) or recommended by me. This list is by no means complete for organic and health food stores around the country, but it is a great start.

VICTORIA

All Organic Life
Balwyn North
Phone: (03) 9857 9930
E-mail: contact@allorganiclife.com.au

Altona North Organics
Altona North
Phone: (03) 9391 3282
Fax: (03) 9391 1990

Angelo's Organic & Biodynamic Natureland
Blackburn
Phone: (03) 9877 3030

B-COZ Restaurant
Hawthorn East
Phone: (03) 9882 7889
Fax: (03) 9882 7898
E-mail: rod@bcoz.com.au
Web: www.bcoz.com.au

Camberwell Fruit Basket
Camberwell
Phone: (03) 9813 1736
Fax: (03) 9383 1402
E-mail:
camberwellfruitbasket@yahoo.com.au

Ceres Organic Farm
Brunswick
Phone: (03) 9387 2609
Fax: (03) 9381 1844
E-mail: chris@ceres.org.au

Cheltenham Organic Store
Cheltenham
Phone: (03) 9583 8754
Fax: (03) 9583 4987

Deliciously Organic
Clifton Hill
Phone: (03) 9489 0051
Fax: (03) 9489 0106
E-mail: info@dostore.com.au

Don't Panic It's Organic
Mt Eliza
Phone: (03) 9775 2024
Fax: (03) 9775 2024

Eastfield Natural Foods
Croydon South
Phone: (03) 9723 0257
Fax: (03) 9723 1144

Geelong's Wholefoods
Geelong
Phone: (03) 5221 5421
Fax: (03) 5221 5429

Get Real Organics
Yarrambat
Phone: (03) 9434 6233
Fax: (03) 9436 1849
E-mail:
getrealorganics@optusnet.com.au

Joe's Organic Market
Alphington
Phone: (03) 9499 4646
Fax: (03) 9499 4646
E-mail: joe@joesorganic.com
Web: www.joesorganic.com

Kew Organics
Kew
Phone: (03) 9852 8955
Fax: (03) 9852 8399

Organic Central
Templestowe
Phone: (03) 9846 5551
Fax: (03) 9846 5501
E-mail: mirok@aanet.com.au

Organic Indulgence
Pascoe Vale South
Phone: (03) 9384 3006
Fax: (03) 9386 2404
E-mail: scriff@iprimus.com.au

Organically Grown
Malvern
Phone: (03) 9500 9796

Organics at the Market
Eaglemont
Phone: (03) 9326 5563
Fax: (03) 9440 9646
E-mail: oatm@optusnet.com.au

Plump Organic Grocery
Yarraville
Phone: (03) 9687 6422
Fax: (03) 9687 6322
E-mail: shop@plump.com.au

Rhubarb Rhubarb Organics
Preston
Phone: (03) 9478 7344 [H: Hayden
(03) 9482 6638)]
Fax: (03) 9478 7344

Superfruit Enterprises Pty Ltd
Ivanhoe
Phone: (03) 9497 1055
Fax: (03) 9497 1099

The Fruit Pedallers
Northcote
Phone: (03) 9489 5824

The Organic Larder
Geelong
Phone: (03) 5229 1134
Fax: (03) 5229 1134

The Organic Union
Surrey Hills
Phone: (03) 98901292

Western District Fruit Supply
Warrnambool
Phone: (03) 5562 5667
Fax: (03) 5562 7815

NEW SOUTH WALES

Be Organic
Cromer Heights
Phone: (02) 9982 8630 Home
Fax: (02) 9982 8630
E-mail: enquiry@beorganic.com.au

Kellyville Pizzeria
West Ryde
Phone: (02) 9874 1559
Fax: (02) 9874 1559
E-mail: dmourani@hotmail.com

Lettuce Deliver
Rozelle
Phone: (02) 9763 7337
Fax: (02) 9763 7338
E-mail: sales@lettucedeliver.com.au
Web: www.lettucedeliver.com.au

Manly West Organic Market
Cromer Heights
E-mail: info@freshandwild.com.au
Web: www.freshandwild.com.au

More Health Organics
Sydney Market
Phone: (02) 9764 2805
Fax: (02) 9764 2805
E-mail: organics@morehealth.com.au

Newport Health Foods
Newport Beach
Phone: (02) 9997 1238
Fax: (02) 9979 5731
E-mail: patrickpollnow@hotmail.com

Organic Feast
East Maitland
Phone: (02) 4934 7351
Fax: (02) 4934 7070
E-mail: sales@organicfeast.com.au

Organic Fresh Pty Ltd
Homebush
Phone: 1300 881 161
Fax: 1300 881 171
E-mail: info@theorganicgrocer.com.au

Singleton Organics
Singleton
Phone: (02) 6572 3444
Fax: (02) 6572 3444
E-mail: terrgroc@bigpond.net.au

The Health Emporium
Bondi
Phone: (02) 9365 6008
Fax: (02) 9300 9330
E-mail: thebondi@bigpond.net.au

The Organic Food Network Pty Ltd
Brookvale
Phone: (02) 9938 2364
E-mail: mglanger@bigpond.net.au

ACT

Organic Energy
Canberra
Phone: (02) 6295 6700
[H: (02) 6295 0832]
Fax: (02) 6295 6701
E-mail: karenmedbury@hotmail.com

SOUTH AUSTRALIA

Central Organics
Adelaide
Phone: (08) 8211 8526
E-mail: oulianoff@internode.com.au

Fast Life Organic
Adelaide
Phone: (08) 8223 3187
Fax: (08) 8223 3387
E-mail: food@fastlifeorganic.com
Web: www.fastlifeorganic.com

Feast Fine Foods & The Chop Shop
Kent Town
Phone: (08) 8132 1355
Fax: (08) 8132 1366
E-mail: richard@rgfm.com.au

Goodlife Modern Organic Pizza
Adelaide
Phone: (08) 8223 2618
Fax: (08) 8223 2101
E-mail: martingreenrod@adam.com.au
Web: www.goodlifepizza.com

WESTERN AUSTRALIA

Organic Foods Australia
Malaga
Phone: (08) 9248 4506
E-mail: organicfoods@hotmail.com

Wembly Supa IGA
Wembley
Phone: (08) 9387 9500
Fax: (08) 9383 7011
E-mail:
vince@dewsonswembley.com.au

QUEENSLAND

Sun and Earth Whole Foods
New Farm
Phone: (07) 3358 2299
Fax: (07) 3358 2199
E-mail: sunandearth@iprimus.com.au

The Organic Shed
Mt Pleasant
Phone: (07) 4954 0820
Fax: (07) 4954 0708
E-mail: organic@mackay.net.au

The Natural Food Store
352 Mons Road
Forest Glen
Phone: (07) 5445 6440
Web: www.thenaturalfoodstore.com.au

Nude Food Organics
3–5 Burns Avenue
Kawana
Phone: (07) 5444 5552
E-mail:
nudefoodorganics@bigpond.com.au

Mrs. Flannery's Natural Grocers
Central One, 45 Plaza Parade
Maroochydore
Phone: (07) 5479 3522
E-mail:
maroochydore@mrsflannerys.com.au

The Organic Apple
Marcoola
Phone: (07) 5448 7709
Fax: (07) 5448 7707
E-mail: organic-apple@netspace.net.au

Wray Organic – Broadbeach
Broadbeach
Phone: (07) 5592 1007
Web: www.wrayorganic.com.au

Wray Organic – Indooroopilly
Indooroopilly
Phone: (07) 3871 3411
Web: www.wrayorganic.com.au

Wray Organic – Newmarket
Newmarket
Phone: (07) 3356 0444
Web: www.wrayorganic.com.au

Wray Organic – Palm Beach
Palm Beach
Phone: (07) 5576 7111
Web: www.wrayorganic.com.au

FURTHER INFORMATION

For more information regarding the
growth or export of organic or
biodynamic produce, contact:

AQIS Organic Program

**Program Management and
Operations:**
+61 2 6271 6638 or +61 2 6272 5217

Policy and Market Access:
+61 2 6272 3509
Fax: +61 2 6272 3238
E-mail: organic@aqis.gov.au

OR
Contact one of the Approved Certifying
Organisations listed below:

Australian Certified Organic
PO Box 530 Chermside 4032
Level 1, 766 Gympie Rd Chermside
4032
Contact: Paul Dargusch or
Akiko Nicholls
Phone: +61 7 3350 5706
Fax: +61 7 3350 5996
E-mail: info@australianorganic.com.au
Web: www.australianorganic.com.au

Bio-Dynamic Research Institute
Post Office Powelltown 3797
Main Rd Powelltown 3797
Contact: Frances Porter or
Alex Podolinsky
Phone: +61 3 5966 7333
Fax: +61 3 5966 7433
Web: www.demeter.org.au

National Association for Sustainable Agriculture Australia
Post Office Box 768 Stirling 5152
Unit 7, 3 Mount Baker Rd Stirling 5152
Contact: Lyn Austin or George Devrell
Phone: +61 8 8370 8455
Fax: +61 8 8370 8381
E-mail: enquiries@nasaa.com.au
Web: www.nasaa.com.au

OGA Certified Pty Ltd
Post Office Box 6171 Sth Lismore 2480
Southern Cross University Crawford Rd
Lismore 2480
Contact: Debbie Holley or
Howard Rubin
Phone: +61 2 6622 0100
Fax: +61 2 6622 0900
E-mail: oga@nrg.com.au
Web: www.organicgrowers.org.au

Organic Food Chain
PO Box 2390 Toowoomba, Qld 4350
Lamascotte Kelvinhough Boodua Rd
Boodua via Oakey 4401
Contact: Marg Will or Ivy Inwood
Phone: +61 7 4637 2600
Fax: +61 7 4696 7689
E-mail: ofc@organicfoodchain.com.au
Web: www.organicfoodchain.com.au

Safe Food Production Queensland
PO Box 440 Spring Hill, Qld 4004
12 Helen St Newstead, Qld 4006
Contact: Paula Seal, Kerry Bell or
Phil Pond

Phone: +61 7 3253 9800 or
1800 300 815
Fax: +61 7 3253 9824
E-mail: info@safefood.qld.gov.au
Web: www.safefood.qld.gov.au

Tasmanian Organic-dynamic Producers
PO Box 434 Mowbray Heights, Tas 7248
197 Wilks Road Lorinna 7306
Contact: Julie Page or Joe Gretschmann
Phone: +61 3 6363 5162 or
mobile 0427 613 697
Fax: +61 3 6363 5162
E-mail: tas_organicdynamic@yahoo.com
Web: n/a

Other References

For a guide to the symbols of these
organisations please refer to the
website: www.changinghabits.com.au

Greenpeace True Food Guide – for GM-
free foods:
http://sites.greenpeace.org.au/true-
food/guide2.html

Rapadura Sugar Victorian Distributor
Organic Times Pty Ltd.
Factory 11/22 Bridge St
Eltham, Vic 3095
Phone: +61 3 9439 7799
Fax: +61 3 9439 5155
E-mail: info@organictimes.com.au

Rapadura Sugar NSW/Qld Distributor
Gio's Organic
43 Wollumbin St
Murwillumbah, NSW 2484
Phone: +61 2 6672 2715
Fax: +61 2 6672 6649
E-mail:
Freshwholefood@westnet.com.au

INDEX

Need a dynamic, informative and entertaining speaker guaranteed to inspire the audience at your next business or networking function?

Cyndi O'Meara is passionate and knowledgeable about health issues and uses her education and experience to help others enjoy longer, healthier lives.

Her unique down-to-earth approach challenges and encourages people to eliminate unhealthy habits and has inspired thousands to make smarter choices about the food they choose to put into their body. Cyndi confronts her audiences with new truths and empowers them to make long lasting changes in simple and achievable steps.

Named Sunshine Coast Businesswoman of the Year in 2003, Cyndi is available for a limited number of speaking engagements each year. If you are interested in booking Cyndi as a keynote speaker for your next conference or business event, contact *Changing Habits, Changing Lives* through www.changinghabits.com.au